AF480735

THE PATH TO DEFEAT CANCER

Revolutionary AI-Powered Early Cancer Detection

Dr. Stanley SY Chen

DEDICATION

This book is dedicated to all the people who seek to minimize the risk of cancer by sharing an actionable plan for proactive systemic early detection to catch cancer at early, curable stages.

TABLE OF CONTENTS

PREFACE

Cancer remains one of the most feared and deadly diseases, affecting every family and touching everyone's life, either directly or indirectly. Countless individuals, including myself, are keenly aware of and concerned about the risk of cancer. Cancer can grow silently and go unnoticed in the body until it's too late, even when we feel fit, live healthy lifestyles, and have no family history.

What can we do to eliminate or drastically reduce our cancer risk? What is the best path forward to defeat cancer? This book aims to address these crucial questions.

The book is organized into three parts:

The Cancer Crisis — Why Is Cancer Still So Prevalent and Deadly? In this part, I review and scrutinize the latest breakthroughs and ongoing challenges in cancer treatment and prevention. I then address the following questions:

- Why is late-stage cancer still largely incurable?

- Why is prevention still so ineffective?

- Why is early detection so challenging?

The Hope — Breakthrough Technologies That Can Detect Most Cancers Early with a Single Test.

In the second part, I explore emerging, revolutionary AI-powered systemic detection tests that can catch most cancers early. I especially examine the scientific basis, potential, and pitfalls of these cutting-edge detection technologies:

- How can Multi-Cancer Early Detection (MCED) tests detect the signals of most cancer types with a single blood test?

- How can whole-body MRI detect early cancer lesions and other medical conditions before symptoms appear?

- How is AI transforming systemic early cancer detection by integrating with these cutting-edge detection technologies?

The Guide — Taking Action to Catch Most Cancers Early and Save Lives.

In the last part, I present a practical plan for systemic early detection across the entire body as individual-driven, proactive health care.

After reading this book, you will gain a clear understanding of both the latest advancements and the ongoing challenges in cancer treatment, prevention, and early detection.

You'll understand the potential and pitfalls of groundbreaking technologies like MCED blood tests and whole-body MRI scans in detecting most cancers at their earliest stages.

Armed with this knowledge, you'll be empowered to make informed, science-based decisions about when and how to adopt these innovative tests to catch most cancers early, potentially saving lives.

PART I

The Cancer Crisis

Why Is Cancer Still So Prevalent and Deadly?

Introduction: Still the Most Fearful Disease

CHAPTER ONE

Throughout human history, few adversaries have proven as formidable as cancer. It is a tale as old as humanity, a saga of struggle and resilience spanning centuries. This narrative begins in the dusty tomes of ancient Egypt, where the first whispers of this shadowy enemy were recorded around the Pyramid Age (around 3000-2500 BC) in the Edwin Smith Papyrus, an ancient Egyptian medical text. The ancient Greeks, led by the venerable Hippocrates (450-380 BC), called it "carcinos," meaning crab—a chilling metaphor for how this disease scuttles through the body, its tendrils grasping at life itself.

Siddhartha Mukherjee aptly describes cancer as the "emperor of all maladies" in his seminal work, "The Emperor of All Maladies: A Biography of Cancer." It is not just one villain but a legion, a rogue's gallery of diseases, each with its own sinister method of unleashing chaos within the body. These cellular mutineers multiply unchecked, possessing an insidious ability to travel and metastasize. Like seeds carried on a bitter wind, they take root in distant parts, sprouting new tumors and creating nascent ruinous grooves.

The complexity of this foe is staggering. Cancer can manifest anywhere, wearing a different face in each encounter. Sometimes, it lurks in the lungs; other times, it besieges the breast or invades the blood. Each type of cancer is a unique puzzle with cryptic clues and shifting solutions. As if these challenges weren't enough, cancer exploits our very genes and environment against us, turning personal habits and inherited traits into unwitting accomplices.

From Fear to a Call for Action

In the utopia of one's mind, countless dreams unfold for oneself and loved ones. Yet, a lurking horror in the reality of our world threatens to disrupt this serene vision. Cancer, often hailed as the unpredicted, undefeated emperor of maladies, is a lifelong curse affecting millions globally. It can emerge in any part of the body, infiltrating healthy tissues and disrupting their normal functions.

The enigma of cancer has baffled and eluded scientists for centuries. It strikes indiscriminately, showing no mercy to its victims. The devastation it causes and the heartbreak of losing loved ones have driven researchers and physicians to dedicate their lives to understanding and eradicating this scourge. Cancer can invade any part of the body, slowly deteriorating vital organs, making its diagnosis deadly frightening. Yet, the indomitable spirit of medical professionals and researchers shines brightly as they tirelessly work to end this relentless nightmare. As Mukherjee eloquently puts it, "The quest for a cure for cancer is a quintessential human endeavor—a drive to understand and ultimately transcend our biological limitations." This quest took flight in the 19th century when advances in surgery, anesthesia, and antiseptics allowed doctors to excise tumors with better safety and precision. The 20th century saw an explosion of progress: radiation to burn away cancer cells, chemotherapy to poison them, and, in recent times, therapies that turn our own immune systems into cancer-hunting champions.

Yet, beyond the laboratories and operating rooms beats a universal heart that longs for a world unburdened by this scourge. Mukherjee captures this dream by writing that cancer is "the scrappy, surreptitious, rule-breaking fragment of our humanity." To dream of curing it is to dream of taming that wild, destructive part of ourselves and rewriting the rules of our own biology.

Imagine that world. A world where no child knows the fear of losing a parent too soon, where no lover has to say goodbye prematurely. This isn't just a medical aspiration; it's a testament to the resilience of the human spirit and a beacon of hope that refuses to be extinguished. It's a flame passed from one generation to the next, fueled by loss, love, and an unyielding belief in a better tomorrow.

This is the story of cancer and humanity—a tale of an ancient, adaptable foe and a species that refuses to bow down. It's a narrative of struggle, incremental victories, and an enduring dream. A dream that one day, in the not-too-distant future, we will turn the final page on cancer's grim history and begin a new chapter—one where life, uninterrupted by this malady, can flourish in all its vibrant glory and peace.

In the grand narrative of humanity's battle against cancer, a thread of extraordinary resilience stands out, intricately woven by Mary Lasker. Her story is not one of laboratories and microscopes but of boardrooms and corridors of power, where she wielded influence with the precision of a scalpel, steadfast in her mission to carve out a future free from cancer's shadow.

Mary Lasker was not a scientist donning a white coat and peering into cellular chaos. She was a warrior in high heels, a philanthropist whose battleground was the marble halls of Washington, DC. In the late 1960s, while the nation's eyes were fixed on the stars, Lasker's focus was on an enemy within. She saw cancer not as an inevitable fate but as a foe that could be defeated with the full force of American ingenuity and resources.

With the zeal of a general rallying her troops, Lasker founded the Citizens Committee for the Conquest of Cancer. This was no ordinary committee; it was a war council. She gathered luminaries from science, medicine, and public life, each a beacon of hope. Together, they shared a bold, urgent vision: to harness the federal government's vast resources in a coordinated assault on cancer.

Their battle cry came in December 1969, not through a rousing speech but a full-page advertisement in the Washington Post. It was Lasker's masterstroke, a public declaration of war against an enemy that had waged a silent, insidious campaign against humanity for too long. The advertisement was a clarion call; its ink-stained words targeted the hearts of policymakers and the public alike.

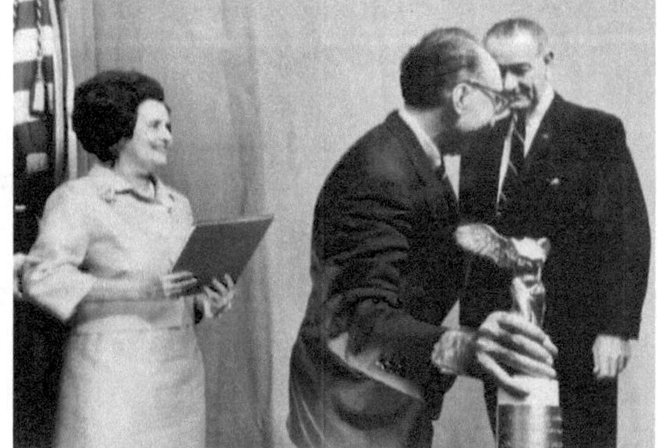

Source: Lasker Foundation

"We are losing the War on Cancer," the ad proclaimed, delivering a stark jolt to the national consciousness. It painted cancer not merely as a medical issue but as a scourge that stole loved ones and drained the nation's resources. Lasker and her committee argued that just as America had committed to planting a flag on the moon, it must now pledge its wealth, intellect, and will to achieving victory over cancer.

This was no plea for pity or charity. It was a demand for action, a call to redirect the nation's focus from the vastness of space to the intricate battlefields within our bodies. The message was clear: with the same determination that fueled rockets and built lunar modules, America could, and must, conquer cancer. The cost of inaction, they warned, was measured not just in dollars but in irreplaceable human lives.

Lasker's campaign was a testament to the power of a single voice, amplified by conviction and strategy. Her story reminds us that the fight against cancer is waged not only in laboratories but also in the hearts and minds of those who dare to envision a world where this enemy is finally irrevocably defeated. It's a narrative of courage, not just of those who face cancer in hospital beds but of those who confront bureaucracy and apathy to make that vision a reality.

In the annals of this ongoing war, Mary Lasker stands as a general whose weapons were words, whose strategy was persuasion, and whose ultimate victory would be measured in lives saved and families kept whole. Her legacy on the war on cancer reminds us that in the battle against cancer, every voice raised in advocacy and every dollar committed to research brings us closer to the day we can finally declare victory.

The Unfulfilled Dream of Finding a Cure

In 1971, President Richard Nixon stood before Congress in his State of the Union address and declared a "war on cancer." His words marked a seismic shift in the national narrative. "The time has come in America," he proclaimed, "when the same kind of concentrated effort that split the atom and took the man to the moon should be turned towards conquering this dread disease." With the stroke of his pen on the National Cancer Act, Nixon marshaled the nation's resources as if preparing for a moon landing, but this time, the target was the insidious enemy within our own body.

The 'War on Cancer' initiative aimed to find a cure for cancer. This initiative revolutionized the approach to cancer by establishing the National Cancer Institute (NCI) and prioritizing cancer research nationally. Significant advancements have been made in treatment, detection, and prevention.

Fast forward forty-five years and another president took up the mantle. In his 2016 State of the Union address, Barack Obama spoke not of war but of a moonshot. "For the loved ones we've all lost, for the families that we can still save," he declared, "let's make America the country that cures cancer once and for all." His words breathed new life into an old dream, entrusting the mission to his vice president, Joe Biden, a man who knew the personal toll of cancer all too well. Biden's cancer moonshot was a mission for a new era.

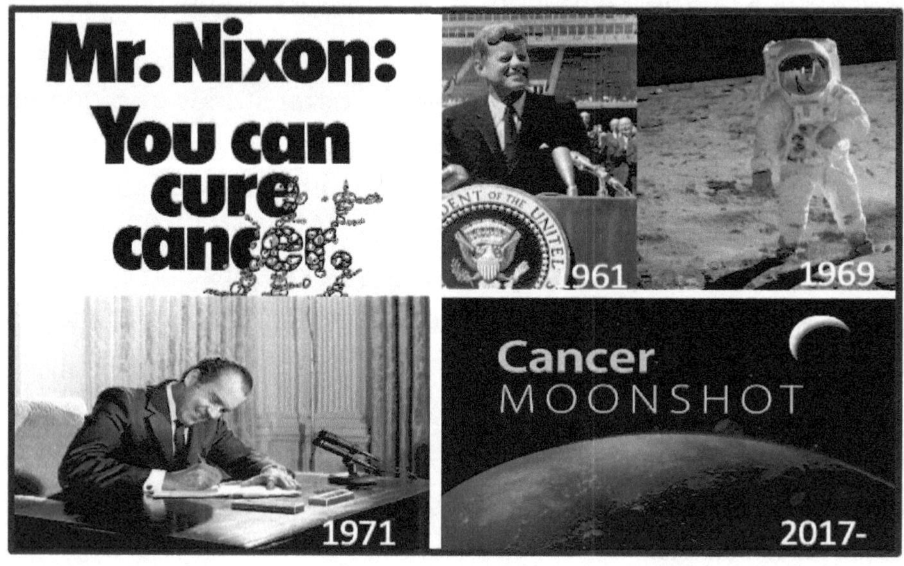

Like the space race that inspired it, it sought to push the boundaries of what was possible. But instead of exploring the cosmos, this journey delved into the microscopic universe of cells and genes. It was a quest to harness the 21st century's most potent tools: vast oceans of big data, intricate maps of the human genome, and the body's own immune system, reprogrammed to hunt down cancer cells.

The legacies of these presidential crusades stretch far beyond their tenures. Nixon's war, despite its military metaphors, planted the seeds of a research ecosystem that would flourish for generations. The ongoing cancer moonshot, with its vision of collaboration, launched a new age of innovation where breakthroughs could come from anywhere, fueled by shared knowledge and a common purpose.

Since 1991, the overall cancer death rate in the US has decreased by 29%, with substantial rate reductions observed across the four most common cancers: lung, colorectal, breast, and prostate, although the total number of cancer cases and deaths still rises. These improvements are attributed to a combination of reduced smoking rates, enhanced screening practices, and better treatment options. Despite these advancements, the incidence of cancer still rises, primarily due to the aging population and an increase in lifestyle-related risk factors such as obesity.

For all these advances, the main goal—a cure for cancer—remains elusive. No magic bullet has been found, and cancer's shadow still falls across hospital beds and family dinners, a grim reminder of the arduous journey ahead.

Feeling Vulnerable and Powerless

In the delicate tapestry of modern human life, a malevolent monster still looms that can snag any life and unravel any future. This monster is cancer, and its insidious nature was somberly revealed when it entangled itself in the life of Princess Kate of Britain, a vibrant young woman who

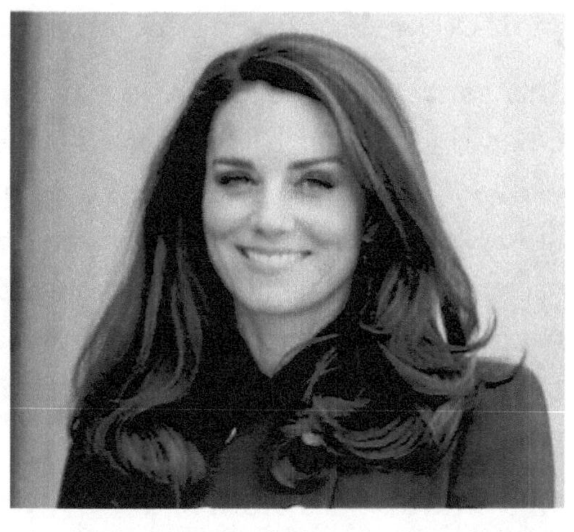

epitomized health. Her diagnosis sent ripples through the world, a stark reminder that this disease respects neither those who wield the crown nor those who bow before it. Susan Wojcicki, a trailblazing figure in Silicon Valley and former CEO of YouTube, sadly passed away on August 9, 2024, at 56, following a two-year battle with lung cancer. Despite having access to extensive resources and cutting-edge medical treatments, her passing highlights the relentless impact of cancer. As a prominent tech executive with ties to some of the world's leading medical institutions, Wojcicki had access to state-of-the-art treatments and clinical trials. Nonetheless, her death is a poignant reminder that cancer remains a formidable adversary, capable of taking lives irrespective of wealth, status, or access to advanced healthcare.

Cancer's indiscriminate cruelty is a tale I know all too well. It's etched in the empty chairs at my dinner table, in the silence where once there was laughter. Two longtime friends, who were in their fifties and seemingly in vibrant health, discovered only later that their bodies had been silently ravaged by metastasized cancer. Under the excellent care and guardianship of the world's most eminent physicians in Johns Hopkins Hospital and Penn Medicine, they waged valiant but ultimately losing battles. Like countless others, their stories are bitter testaments to the limits of even the most advanced medical treatments.

This sense of vulnerability is certainly not mine alone. In bustling cities and quaint towns across America and far beyond, people whisper their fears and share the sense of vulnerability I have felt. Surveys echo with a common dread: the fear of cancer's shadow falling across their lives. Yet, alongside this fear is a more insidious emotion: powerlessness. It's as if we stand on the shore, knowing a tsunami approaches and will crash upon us, yet feeling utterly unable to escape.

This randomness creates a sense of vulnerability and uncertainty, as even the healthiest individuals may find themselves battling this insidious disease. "Cancer is a disease that doesn't discriminate. It doesn't care if you're rich or poor, black or white, young or old.", said Kathy Bates, an actress who was diagnosed with ovarian cancer in 2003 and then breast cancer in 2012.

However, we are not entirely without weapons. The shield of a healthy lifestyle—a diet rich in nature's bounty, regular exercise, and the wisdom to shun tobacco—can reduce our risk. Yet, the cruel twist in cancer's tale lies: even the most fortified citadel can fall to its long-term siege.

Within the very clockwork of our cells lies a traitor. As cells divide and multiply—a process as natural as the rising sun—errors can creep in. These random mutations, these genetic misprints, can transform a loyal cell into a rogue. It's a lottery no one wants to win, a game of cellular roulette where the stakes are life itself. This element of chance, this roll of the biological dice, is why cancer can strike down a vibrant marathon runner as well as a weathered elderly person.

Confronted by such unpredictability and deadly whims, one cannot help but feel vulnerable and fearful. Yet, the aspiration to conquer cancer remains undiminished. This dream is woven from the tears of those who have endured losses, the bravery of those who persist in their fight, and the unyielding hope that, in the future radiant with promise, the word 'cancer' will signify nothing more than a tamed adversary, devoid of its former terror.

A Bright New Path Forward Owing to Detection Technology Breakthroughs

Buoyed by the hope for its defeat and haunted by the dread of this adversary, we are compelled to ask how we can defeat this formidable foe should a cure continue to elude us.

It is apparent to me that incremental advances in targeted therapy, immunotherapy, and their combinations are unlikely to defeat this clever, adaptable enemy. This realization comes from more than thirty years of my dedicated effort in the fight against cancer, where the foe is an ever-shifting array of uncontrolled cells, mutating and proliferating with daunting unpredictability.

My battlegrounds have been the research facilities and hospitals of America's esteemed medical centers, starting from the Dana-Farber Cancer Institute and Harvard Medical School to the Texas Medical Center in Houston, and the University of Southern California Medical Center. In this book, I invite you to traverse the complex pathways of our battle against cancer, observing both the victories and challenges we face. Together, we will explore the cutting-edge advances that have transformed fatal prognoses into tales of endurance, the vigilant guardians of early detection, and the sturdy ramparts of prevention. This book is more than a mere compendium of facts; it is a guide meticulously charted with extensive research findings and marked by the profound sentiments of both despair and hope.

Then, as we gaze towards the horizon, the dawn of a new era in the fight against cancer unfolds before us, illuminated by groundbreaking advances in cancer detection technologies. Pathways once veiled in darkness now gleam brightly, charting our course forward.

On the cusp of transformative breakthroughs, we stand poised to venture into new territories once relegated to the realm of science fiction. Envision a world where the early detection of cancer is as straightforward as a routine blood test and a brief imaging scan long before it manifests any symptoms, all enabled by the sophisticated capabilities of rapidly advancing artificial intelligence (AI). These cutting-edge technologies, as exemplified by blood circulating tumor DNA (ctDNA) detection and whole-body magnetic resonance imaging (MRI), are evolving from initial conceptualizations to proven clinical applications, gradually transitioning into the sphere of daily medical practice. These preventive systemic screening tests for detecting most cancer types, through AI-powered early detection of the whole body, are heralding a new era in the battle against cancer, promising transformative breakthroughs.

Let us embark on a grand tour of the dynamic and ever-evolving battlefield in the fight against cancer, as we forge innovative paths to defeat this formidable and elusive adversary by harnessing AI-powered systemic early detection to catch most types of cancer at early, curable stages.

The Enduring Challenge of Finding a Cure

CHAPTER TWO

"When we long for life without difficulties, remind us that oaks grow strong in contrary winds and diamonds are made under pressure."
Peter Marshall

How can we find a cure for advanced cancer?

Hope is a mosaic, intricately pieced together from the threads of human ingenuity and buoyant spirits. The plight faced by millions diagnosed with cancer each year, their battle against this formidable disease, and their resilience create a collective mission. The universal aspiration to find a cure for cancer resonates deeply across humanity.

The 1980s and 1990s were eras of immense enthusiasm and optimism among researchers and physicians in seeking a cure for cancer—a hope grounded in technological advances. Emerging, groundbreaking technologies in antibody engineering, genetic engineering, and automated DNA sequencing for human genome projects opened up boundless possibilities for innovative cancer treatments.

My journey in the fight against cancer began in 1991 at the Dana-Farber Cancer Institute and the Department of Pathology at Harvard Medical School. As a fellow armed with medical knowledge and biotechnology expertise, I was driven by a passionate commitment to finding a cure. Since 1994, I have led my interdisciplinary research team, composed of physicians, researchers, medical students, and graduate students, to develop innovative therapies. We have harnessed the power of antibody and genetic engineering to create a range of innovative therapies against cancer and HIV. Our efforts include developing novel intrabodies that block oncoproteins within cancer cells, tumor vaccines that activate the immune system against cancer, antibody-fusion proteins that deliver toxic payloads to tumors, and CAR T cell therapy.

Our journey has been arduous, marked by advances as well as setbacks that obstructed our path. Yet, each hurdle only strengthened our resolve, propelling us forward with renewed vigor. Today, as a seasoned veteran in the fight against cancer, I, along with countless physicians and researchers, take immense pride in the tremendous strides we have made.

The FDA has approved over 200 cancer drugs since 2010, many of which are targeted therapies that attack specific genetic mutations in cancer cells. In addition to targeted therapies, immunotherapies have transformed the cancer treatment landscape. By harnessing the power of our own immune system to fight cancer, these groundbreaking treatments have shown remarkable success in treating previously untreatable cancers. From checkpoint inhibitors that release the brakes on the immune system to CAR T cell therapy that reprograms a patient's immune cells, these treatments have revolutionized how we treat cancer, resulting in improved survival rates and quality of life for patients. These advances have reinvigorated the spirits of physicians and researchers alike. The pace of progress in cancer therapeutics has been breathtaking.

Let us take a moment to review and celebrate the monumental advances in our journey of finding a cure for cancer, achieved by countless dedicated and talented physicians and scientists in the US and around the world.

Advances in Cancer Treatment

Cancer treatment integrates various approaches: surgery, radiotherapy, chemotherapy, targeted therapy, and immunotherapy. Surgical techniques have evolved dramatically, now offering unprecedented precision and minimal invasiveness to remove cancerous tissue. Robotic tools and advanced imaging technologies enable surgeons to visualize tumors with exceptional clarity, allowing for more accurate surgery. Radiation therapy uses high-energy radiation to eliminate cancer cells. Techniques such as intensity-modulated radiation therapy precisely target tumors while sparing surrounding healthy tissues, thereby reducing side effects. Chemotherapy involves the use of chemical drugs to destroy dividing cancer cells.

The advent of targeted therapies marks a significant milestone in cancer treatment. These therapies focus on malignant cells while sparing healthy tissues, improving treatment outcomes, and minimizing side effects. Additionally, immunotherapy has revolutionized cancer care by leveraging the body's immune system to combat cancer. This includes promising approaches such as checkpoint inhibitors, CAR T cell therapy, and cancer vaccines, which are at the forefront of contemporary research.

Here, I will highlight the vast array of advanced cancer drugs in the arsenal, so you, not being in the field of oncology or a medical professional, will know where physicians and scientists have been focusing their efforts, resources, and energy in the fight against cancer. Of course, you don't need to know the details of these cutting-edge treatments; you can simply scan through the contents to grasp the landscape of advanced cancer therapies that are available and in development.

Arsenal of Advanced Cancer Drugs:

Targeted Therapy:
- **Small Molecule Inhibitors**
  - **Kinase inhibitors**
  - **Other inhibitors**
- **Antibodies:**
  - **Antibodies (naked, mono-specific)**
  - **Bi-specific/multi-specific antibodies**
  - **Bi-specific T-cell engagers (BiTEs)**
  - **Antibody-drug conjugates (ADCs)**

Immunotherapy:
- **Immune Checkpoint Blockade**
- **CAR T Cell Therapy**
- **Tumor-Infiltrating Lymphocyte (TIL) Therapy**
- **Tumor Vaccine**

Targeted Therapy with Small Molecule Inhibitors

Scientists and physicians have dreamed of having a therapy that would be so specific in its approach that it would be able to hit cancer while staying clear of the healthy tissues. This dream of a 'magic bullet' against cancer was first launched in the early 1900s by Paul Ehrlich, and it took almost a century for the potential of this dream to be realized.

In the 1970s, scientists realized that estrogen is related to some forms of breast cancer. Drugs such as tamoxifen can block the hormone receptors and starve the tumors of their fuel. This was the beginning of targeted therapy against cancer.

Important advancements in genetics and biotechnology in the 1980s and 90s cracked open cancer's molecular blueprint. Scientists learned specific genetic mutations and disrupted pathways that turned normal cells into uncontrolled cancerous ones. These discoveries led to the development of 'small molecule inhibitors' targeting specific disrupted pathways in cancer cells.

The Targeted Drug Gleevec: A Paradigm Shift

The groundbreaking example of this strategy was the FDA's approval of imatinib (Gleevec) for chronic myeloid leukemia in 2001. Imatinib was the first of these agents, which targets the BCR-ABL tyrosine kinase, the molecular driving force for this cancer. Its use led to a new age of targeted therapies with superior specificity and less toxicity than chemotherapy agents.

Since then, numerous small molecule "magic bullets" have been synthesized, where each molecule is designed to kill cancer by targeting a specific pathway responsible for the uncontrolled growth of cancer cells. A large number of small molecule inhibitors have been approved by the FDA for cancer treatment and are highlighted here.

Protein Kinase Inhibitors

Protein kinases play a crucial role in cancer growth and have become important targets for cancer therapy. Protein kinases are enzymes that regulate critical cellular functions by adding phosphate groups to other proteins, a process called phosphorylation. In cancer, many kinases become dysregulated due to mutations or overexpression, leading to uncontrolled cell growth, proliferation, and survival. Kinase inhibitors have emerged as a major class of targeted cancer therapies. They work by blocking the activity of specific kinases that are overactive in cancer cells. Most kinase inhibitors are small molecules competing with ATP to bind to the kinase's active site. Inhibitors can target single kinases or multiple related kinases. Here are the examples of these protein kinase inhibitors:

- Tyrosine Kinase Inhibitors (TKIs): Drugs such as imatinib, erlotinib, and gefitinib are designed to attach to the ATP-binding site of tyrosine kinases, thereby preventing their activation and subsequent signaling cascades that promote cancer cell proliferation. These inhibitors have been particularly effective in treating cancers like chronic myeloid leukemia and non-small cell lung cancer (NSCLC).

- BCR-ABL Inhibitors: Gleevec, Dasatinib, Nilotinib, and Ponatinib are used primarily for CML and acute lymphoblastic leukemia. These inhibitors target the BCR-ABL fusion protein, a product of a chromosomal translocation that causes these leukemias.

- EGFR Inhibitors: Gefitinib (Iressa), Erlotinib, and Osimertinib target the epidermal growth factor receptor (EGFR), which is often mutated in NSCLC, providing a critical therapeutic option for patients with these mutations.

- ALK/ROS1 Inhibitors: Crizotinib, Ceritinib, Alectinib, and Brigatinib target rearrangements in the ALK and ROS1 genes, also common in subsets of NSCLC patients, offering tailored treatments for patients with these mutations.

Other Notable Inhibitors

In addition to protein kinase inhibitors, small molecule inhibitors have been developed to target other processes responsible for the uncontrolled growth of cancer cells. Here are the examples of these inhibitors:

- Proteasome Inhibitors: Bortezomib is a notable example that inhibits the proteasome's function, causing a lethal buildup of cellular waste in cancer cells, particularly effective in multiple myeloma.

- Angiogenesis Inhibitors: Sunitinib and Sorafenib inhibit vascular endothelial growth factor receptors (VEGFRs), disrupting the blood supply to tumors and effectively starving them of necessary nutrients and oxygen.

- PARP Inhibitors: PARP (Poly ADP-Ribose Polymerase) is a class of nuclear enzymes that play a crucial role in DNA damage detection and repair, contributing to the maintenance of genomic stability. Drugs like Olaparib, Rucaparib, and Niraparib exploit synthetic lethality in cancers with defective DNA repair mechanisms, such as BRCA-mutated breast and ovarian cancers. By inhibiting PARP, these drugs prevent cancer cells from repairing DNA damage, leading to cell death.

- mTOR Inhibitors: mTOR (mammalian target of rapamycin) is a key protein kinase that plays a critical role in cancer development and progression. mTOR is a serine/threonine kinase that regulates fundamental cellular processes, including cell growth, proliferation, survival, protein synthesis, and metabolism. The mTOR signaling pathway is frequently dysregulated in various types of human cancers. It is estimated to be aberrantly overactivated in more than 70% of cancers. Everolimus and Temsirolimus inhibit the mTOR pathway, which is critical for cell growth and metabolism, providing therapeutic benefits in renal cell carcinoma and breast cancer.

- CDK4/6 Inhibitors: Palbociclib, Ribociclib, and Abemaciclib target cyclin-dependent kinases 4 and 6, crucial for cell cycle progression and proliferation, offering new treatment avenues for breast cancer.

- IDH Inhibitors: IDH (Isocitrate Dehydrogenase) plays a significant role in cancer cells, particularly when mutated. IDH mutations in cancer cells lead to the production of an oncometabolite, D-2-HG, which drives tumorigenesis. These mutations have become important therapeutic targets in cancer treatment. Ivosidenib and Enasidenib drugs target mutant isocitrate dehydrogenase enzymes in acute myeloid leukemia, presenting novel therapeutic options for these specific genetic mutations.

- Hedgehog Pathway Inhibitor: The Hedgehog signaling pathway plays a significant role in cancer development and progression. In cancer, it often becomes aberrantly activated. Vismodegib targets the Hedgehog signaling pathway, which is implicated in basal cell carcinoma, offering a targeted approach for this skin cancer.

To sum up, small molecule inhibitors have heralded the advance in cancer treatment by providing targeted, less toxic, and effective treatment options. Nevertheless, there are challenges for targeted therapy as cancer can adapt and resist it. Cancer's ability to develop resistance continues to demand increasingly sophisticated combination strategies. Nevertheless, the path pioneered by these molecular magic bullets has irrevocably changed our approach to combating this elusive foe.

Targeted Therapy with Antibodies

Antibody therapy represents a significant advance in cancer treatment. Antibodies can specifically target cancer cells while sparing normal cells, leading to better therapeutic effects and less toxicity.

The concept of antibody therapy can be traced back to the latter half of the nineteenth century. The earliest attempts were made by Emil von Behring and his colleagues, who used antibodies from immunized animals on diphtheria. Emil von Behring, the 'savior of children,' was awarded the first Nobel Prize in Physiology or Medicine in 1901 for developing antibodies against diphtheria toxins. Nevertheless, the antibodies showed promise in treating diseases only in the seventies of the last century.

In 1975, César Milstein and Georges Köhler developed hybridoma technology that made it possible to generate monoclonal antibodies with such specificity previously not imagined. This achievement, decorated with the Nobel Prize in Physiology or

Medicine in 1984, offered a new way to target and destroy cancer cells.

However, a key hurdle of monoclonal antibody therapy is due to the actions of the human immune system against the murine-derived antibodies. This hurdle was surmounted when chimeric and humanized antibodies were developed in the late 1980s and 1990s. Greg Winter was awarded the Nobel Prize in Chemistry in 2018 for his contribution to the phage display of peptides and antibodies for developing humanized antibody therapy. Here is a brief overview of targeted therapy using antibodies and their derivatives:

Antibodies: The FDA's first approval of antibody therapy was muromonab-CD3, a monoclonal antibody for renal transplant rejection in 1986. Cancer-targeting antibodies were subsequently approved for cancer treatment, including rituximab in 1997 targeting CD20 protein in B-cells for non-Hodgkin lymphoma and trastuzumab (Herceptin) in 1998, a potent antibody against HER2-positive breast cancer. Moreover, Cetuximab (Erbitux) was approved in 2004 for head and neck cancer and colorectal cancer through the targeting of EGFR on tumor cells, and Bevacizumab (Avastin) was approved for antiangiogenic therapy through the targeting of VEGF in 2004. These therapies represent precision medicine, with treatment directed toward the cancer cells, improving the therapeutic efficacy and reducing side effects.

In addition to naked antibodies, antibody derivatives have been developed for cancer therapy and are summarized below:

Bispecific/Multispecific Antibodies: Bispecific antibodies are conceived to kill two birds with one stone. This versatile function enables them to carry out numerous tasks like inhibiting two growth factor receptors at once, introducing two varieties of immune cells to the arena of cancer cells, or even placing cytotoxic agents in the tumor cells. Some bispecific antibodies are designed to target and block two crucial signaling pathways relevant to cancer cells.

The FDA has approved several bispecific antibodies for cancer treatment. Rybrevant is an antibody that specifically binds to two receptors, EGFR and MET, and provides a dual blockade on the tumor cell growth signals, which was approved by the FDA in 2021 for treating non-small cell lung cancer. Tecvayli is a BCMA and CD3 bispecific antibody approved 2022 for multiple myeloma. Talquetamab, a bispecific antibody to GPRC5D and CD3, also gained accelerated approval in 2022 to treat multiple myeloma. The bispecific antibody against CD20 and CD3, named mosunetuzumab, is approved for treating follicular lymphoma.

Thus, bispecific and multispecific antibodies represent a new generation of immunotherapy in the fight against cancer.

Bispecific T-Cell Engagers (BiTEs): BiTEs are novel antibodies designed to bind simultaneously to two targets. One part embraces CD3, a protein in T-cells, while the other part hooks a definite antigen on cancer cells. This double locking forms an immunological synapse that triggers T-cells to launch an attack on cancerous cells. Therefore, BiTEs augment the body's defense system, making T-cells lethal for cancers.

The first approval given to BiTE therapy is for blinatumomab. Blinatumomab works against CD19, a protein present in B-cell malignancies, including leukemia as well as lymphoma. Following the success of blinatumomab, a panel of BiTEs, each directed to other cancer antigens, has been developed. Such a candidate includes AMG 330, which targets CD33 in leukemia cells. AMG 330 demonstrates the ability to induce T-cell-mediated cytotoxicity in early-phase clinical trials.

Antibody-Drug Conjugates (ADCs): These innovative therapies are developed as the convergence of targeting the tumor by monoclonal antibodies and toxic chemotherapy drugs. ADCs are effective because they help direct a potent payload right to the cancer cells to spare normal cells affected by conventional chemotherapy.

ADCs are complex molecular constructs composed of three key elements: A monoclonal antibody, a cytotoxic drug, and a protein or small molecule that links the drug to the antibody. The monoclonal antibody functions like a mini-guided missile to target antigens on the cancer cell membrane. The internalization occurs when the ADC binds to its target and is engulfed by the malignant cell by endocytosis. The linker is severed in the cell, and the cytotoxic drug kills by interfering with various cellular processes such as DNA synthesis or microtubules' function in the cancer cell.

One of the first ADCs is trastuzumab emtansine (T-DM1, Kadcyla), targeting the HER2 receptor that is overexpressed in breast cancers. Another ADC is anti-CD30 brentuximab vedotin, intended for the treatment of lymphoma. Brentuximab vedotin has been shown to have a highly potent therapeutic capability. The most recent ADC that entered the market is enfortumab vedotin (Padcev), targeting Nectin-4, an antigen in advanced urothelial cancer. Now, many new ADCs are being developed for cancer treatment.

In summary, the success of antibody-based cancer treatment depends on increasing the ability to target cancer cells, reducing toxicity in healthy cells, and targeting multiple targets, as well as employing the ability to have numerous mechanisms through antibodies, ADCs, and bispecific and multispecific formats. Further studies on improving the most effective designs, target identification, and clinical application strategies will realize their full potential in fighting cancer.

Immunotherapy with Checkpoint Blockade

The advent of immune checkpoint blockade immunotherapy marks a groundbreaking leap forward in cancer treatment.

Immune checkpoints are crucial regulators of the immune system that play a vital role in maintaining self-tolerance and preventing autoimmune responses. Cancer cells can exploit inhibitory checkpoints to evade immune detection and attack, making these pathways critical therapeutic targets in cancer immunotherapy. This innovative approach employs antibodies to block immune checkpoint proteins that cancer cells use to hide from and suppress the immune system. By doing so, it empowers the body's own defenses to fight cancer more effectively.

CTLA4 blockade. Ipilimumab, developed by Bristol-Myers Squibb, was the first immune checkpoint inhibitor approved by the FDA in 2011 for treating advanced melanoma. It is a monoclonal antibody that targets CTLA-4 (Cytotoxic T-Lymphocyte-Associated protein 4), an inhibitory checkpoint molecule expressed on T cells. By blocking CTLA-4, ipilimumab prevents the inhibition of T-cell activation and proliferation, thereby enhancing the immune response against cancer cells. This groundbreaking drug demonstrated significant improvements in overall survival for patients with advanced melanoma. However, due to its mechanism of overaction, ipilimumab can cause immune-related adverse events, including autoimmune reactions in various organs.

PD-1 and PD-L1 blockade. The success of ipilimumab paved the way for developing other checkpoint inhibitors targeting different molecules like PD-1 and PD-L1.

PD-1 (Programmed Cell Death Protein 1) is a receptor protein expressed on the surface of activated T cells, B cells, and myeloid cells. It functions as an "off switch" to help prevent T cells from attacking the body's own cells, thus maintaining self-tolerance and preventing autoimmune responses. PD-L1 (Programmed Death-Ligand 1) is a protein found on the surface of many cell types, including some cancer cells. When PD-L1 binds to PD-1 on T cells, it delivers an inhibitory signal that reduces T cell proliferation and function, effectively suppressing the immune response. This interaction is crucial for regulating the immune system but can be exploited by cancer cells to evade immune detection and destruction.

Many tumor cells overexpress PD-L1 to suppress anti-tumor immune responses, creating an immunosuppressive microenvironment. Blocking the PD-1/PD-L1 interaction with monoclonal antibodies can reactivate T cells, enhancing their ability to recognize and attack cancer cells. This has led to the development of checkpoint inhibitors targeting PD-1 or PD-L1, which have become essential immunotherapy drugs for various cancers. These drugs prevent the inhibitory interaction between PD-1 and PD-L1, thereby boosting the immune system's ability to combat cancer. The understanding and targeting of the PD-1/PD-L1 pathway have resulted in significant advances in cancer treatment, offering new hope for patients with previously untreatable cancers.

In 2014, pembrolizumab (Keytruda) became the first PD-1 inhibitor to be approved for treating advanced melanoma, and the approval was converted to include non-small cell lung cancer in 2015. Other PD-1 inhibitors for cancer treatment include nivolumab (Opdivo) and Libtayo (cemiplimab).

Similarly, PD-L1 inhibitors such as atezolizumab, Tecentriq, durvalumab, Imfinzi, avelumab, and Bavencio have emerged as some of the essential tools in fighting cancer. The immune checkpoint inhibitors approved by the FDA are shown in the table.

These drugs have since become a cornerstone of cancer immunotherapy, showing efficacy across multiple cancer types and leading to durable responses in some patients. The discovery and development of checkpoint inhibitors, including ipilimumab, were groundbreaking achievements in cancer treatment, recognized by the 2018 Nobel Prize in Physiology or Medicine, awarded to James P. Allison and Tasuku Honjo for their work on CTLA-4 and PD-1, respectively.

FDA-Approved Immune Checkpoint Inhibitors

Brand Name	Generic Name	Target	Approved Indications	Approval Year
Yervoy	Ipilimumab	CTLA-4	Melanoma, RCC, Colorectal Cancer, etc.	2011
Keytruda	Pembrolizumab	PD-1	Melanoma, NSCLC, Head and Neck Cancer, etc.	2014
Opdivo	Nivolumab	PD-1	Melanoma, NSCLC, RCC, Hodgkin Lymphoma, etc.	2014
Tecentriq	Atezolizumab	PD-L1	Urothelial Carcinoma, NSCLC, Triple-Negative BC	2016
Bavencio	Avelumab	PD-L1	Merkel Cell Carcinoma, Urothelial Carcinoma	2017
Imfinzi	Durvalumab	PD-L1	Urothelial Carcinoma, NSCLC	2017
Libtayo	Cemiplimab	PD-1	Cutaneous Squamous Cell Carcinoma, NSCLC	2018
Cosela	Trilaciclib	CDK4/6 inhibitor	Small cell lung cancer (to decrease chemotherapy-induced myelosuppression)	2021
Jemperli	Dostarlimab	PD-1	Endometrial Cancer	2021
Zynyz	Retifanlimab	PD-1	Merkel Cell Carcinoma	2023

Blockade of other checkpoints. Nevertheless, not all patients are benefited from PD-1/PD-L1 blockade therapies. Moreover, cancers can become resistant to these therapies. This has provoked a lot of focus on finding other immune checkpoints that can be targeted. The current studies are directed toward discovering and using new immune checkpoints that should add and improve immune checkpoint blockade approaches in the fight against cancer.

A new immune checkpoint protein, also known as lymphocyte activation gene-3 (LAG-3), has a counteracting effect on the activation of T cells. LAG-3 inhibitors are still under clinical trials. Another new checkpoint is the T cell immunoreceptor with Ig and ITIM domains (TIGIT). Often detected with PD-1 on T cells, TIGIT/PD-1 blockade is also under investigation in clinical trials. Based on the first examples, TIGIT inhibition may rejuvenate the exhausted T cells, enhance immune response, and possibly enhance existing PD-1/PD-L1 treatment regimens.

Also, T-cell immunoglobulin and mucin-domain containing-3 (TIM-3) are among the receptors in circulating immune cells. TIM-3 is an exhaustion marker of T cells, and its inhibitor is considered in combination with anti-PD-1/PD-L1 agents. Targeting TIM-3 could affect immune system response in many ways, providing a broader effect.

Combining immune checkpoint inhibitors with other therapies. The primary reason for integrating immune checkpoint inhibitors with other cancer treatments is to multiply the cancer-killing effects of any individual method. This cooperation may be achieved because various treatments influence the tumor and its environment differently. For example, immune checkpoint inhibitors enhance the immune system's capacity to detect and destroy cancer cells; other therapies can decrease the tumor burden or change the tumor microenvironment's identity, rendering it more vulnerable to immunological assault.

Classic chemotherapy that targets dividing cells such as tumor cells has recently been noted to cause immunogenic cell death, setting the tumor to recognition by the immune system. Furthermore, chemotherapy also decreases the number of immune-suppressing cells. Meanwhile, the concept is to synergize chemotherapy with immune checkpoint inhibitors, or more specifically, to pursue a cytotoxic effect together with removing tumor immune checkpoint blockade.

The targeted therapies are specific therapies that focus on interrupting molecular characteristics linked to cancer development and proliferation. When used with immune checkpoint inhibitors, these agents can alter tumor signaling, making the cancer cells susceptible to destruction by the immune system. Radiation therapy kills tumor cells directly and has immunomodulatory effects. It can enhance the exposure of tumor antigens and release cytokines to recruit immune cells to the tumor area from the command. It changes the tumor into an in-situ vaccine. When radiation is used together with immune checkpoint inhibitors, this effect is further enhanced and turned into a systemic therapy.

FDA-Approved Immune Checkpoint Inhibitor Combinations

Combination	Components	Indications	Approval Year
Opdivo + Yervoy	Nivolumab + Ipilimumab	Melanoma, RCC, NSCLC, MSI-H/dMMR Colorectal Cancer	2015
Keytruda + Axitinib	Pembrolizumab + Axitinib	Advanced Renal Cell Carcinoma	2019
Tecentriq + Avastin	Atezolizumab + Bevacizumab	Advanced or Metastatic Hepatocellular Carcinoma	2020
Libtayo + Chemotherapy	Cemiplimab + Chemotherapy	First-line treatment for Advanced NSCLC	2021
Keytruda + Lenvima	Pembrolizumab + Lenvatinib	Endometrial Carcinoma	2021
Opdivo + Cabometyx	Nivolumab + Cabozantinib	Advanced Renal Cell Carcinoma	2021
Imfinzi + Tremelimumab	Durvalumab + Tremelimumab	Unresectable Hepatocellular Carcinoma	2022

The usage of immune checkpoint inhibitors in combination with other cancer treatments is a practical approach that has been adopted in fighting cancer as it has been revealed to increase patients' prognosis. However, as our knowledge of tumor biology, coupled with advances in immunology, continues to be unraveled, these combination approaches will be even more elaborate and, hence, effective in cancer treatment. The table shows the combinations of immune checkpoint inhibitors approved by the FDA.

CAR-T Cell Therapy

In the war against cancer, a wicked new weapon has been devised: armies of the patient's own immune cells, bioengineered to hunt down the cancerous threat. This is the story of CAR T-cell therapy, representing an innovative form of immunotherapy that harnesses the power of a patient's own immune system to fight cancer. CAR T-cell therapy involves modifying a patient's T cells, a type of immune cell, to target and attack cancer cells more effectively.

The process begins by collecting T cells from the patient's blood through apheresis. These cells are then sent to a laboratory, genetically engineered to produce chimeric antigen receptors (CARs) on their surface. These CARs are designed to recognize specific proteins (antigens) on cancer cells.

FDA-Approved CAR T Cell Therapies

Year Approved	Brand Name	Generic Name	Indication	Manufacturer
2017	Kymriah	Tisagenlecleucel	Relapsed or refractory B-cell acute lymphoblastic leukemia (ALL) in patients up to 25 years old	Novartis
2017	Yescarta	Axicabtagene Ciloleucel	Relapsed or refractory large B-cell lymphoma	Kite Pharma/Gilead
2020	Tecartus	Brexucabtagene Autoleucel	Relapsed or refractory mantle cell lymphoma	Kite Pharma/Gilead
2021	Breyanzi	Lisocabtagene Maraleucel	Relapsed or refractory large B-cell lymphoma	Bristol-Myers Squibb
2021	Abecma	Idecabtagene Vicleucel	Relapsed or refractory multiple myeloma	Bristol-Myers Squibb
2022	Carvykti	Ciltacabtagene Autoleucel	Relapsed or refractory multiple myeloma	Janssen/Legend Biotech

Once the modified T cells are produced sufficiently, they are infused into the patient's bloodstream. These CAR T-cells multiply in the body and use their newly engineered receptors to identify and destroy cancer cells. This therapy has shown remarkable success in treating certain types of blood cancers, including some forms of leukemia and lymphoma, particularly in cases where other treatments have failed.

CAR T-cell therapy is currently FDA-approved for treating specific types of relapsed or refractory non-Hodgkin lymphoma, multiple myeloma, and acute lymphoblastic leukemia in both adults and children, as shown in the table. It's available at specialized cancer centers with expertise in cellular therapies.

Mitigating the Toxicities. While CAR T-cell therapy has shown promising results, it can also cause significant side effects, including cytokine release syndrome and neurological toxicities, requiring close monitoring and management by experienced healthcare teams. Cytokine release syndrome (CRS), an inflammatory response, is a serious condition manifesting as a mild flu or severe multi-organ failure. Some measures have been implemented to manage/minimize CRS while enhancing its ability to kill cancer cells. One type involves the administration of antibodies that target and neutralize cytokines that play a key role in the development of CRS, including IL-6.

In collaboration with others, my interdisciplinary research team at the University of Southern California has developed safer CAR T-cell therapies. This safer version of anti-CD19 CAR T cell therapy was designed by re-engineering CAR molecules with reduced signaling intensity. The re-engineered CAR T cells secrete lower amounts of cytokines, synthesize more anti-apoptotic proteins, and have a lower proliferation rate. Yet, their cytotoxicity against malignant cells is not compromised. Based on these results, we embarked on a clinical trial of the re-engineered CAR T cell treatment in B cell lymphoma patients. The results have been promising: achieving impressive anti-lymphoma efficacy without substantial toxicities. Therefore, re-engineered CAR T cells represent a safe and effective therapy (*Nature Medicine*, 2019).

The hurdle of CAR T-Cell Therapy for Solid Tumors. While highly successful in treating certain blood cancers, CAR T-cell therapy faces significant challenges when applied to solid tumors. The primary hurdles include the lack of specific targets unique to solid tumors, tumor heterogeneity leading to antigen escape, and the hostile tumor microenvironment that suppresses CAR T-cell function. Solid tumors often lack clear, unique antigens consistently expressed on cancer cells but not on normal tissues, making it challenging to design CAR T-cells that can effectively target tumor cells without causing significant damage to healthy tissues. Additionally, the diverse cell populations within solid tumors, with varying antigen expression, can result in some cancer cells surviving and continuing to grow, limiting the therapy's effectiveness.

Furthermore, solid tumors create an immunosuppressive microenvironment that can inhibit CAR T-cell function, featuring factors such as hypoxia, acidic pH, and immunosuppressive cells. CAR T-cells often struggle to migrate to and penetrate solid tumors due to physical barriers and a lack of appropriate chemokine signals, limiting their ability to engage with and eliminate cancer cells. The challenging conditions within solid tumors can also lead to rapid CAR T-cell exhaustion, reducing their anti-tumor activity and persistence.

To address these challenges, researchers are exploring strategies, including identifying new tumor-specific antigens, developing multi-target approaches, engineering CAR T-cells to overcome the immunosuppressive tumor microenvironment, and improving T-cell trafficking and infiltration. CRISPR technology is being leveraged to enhance CAR T cell therapy for solid tumors in several innovative ways. By using CRISPR to knock out genes associated with T cell exhaustion, such as PD-1, researchers aim to improve T cell persistence in the hostile tumor microenvironment. The technology also allows editing genes involved in T cell trafficking and migration, potentially enhancing tumor infiltration. While significant obstacles remain, ongoing research and clinical trials are progressing in adapting CAR T-cell therapy for solid tumors, offering hope for future breakthroughs.

Tumor-Infiltrating Lymphocyte (TIL) Therapy

In the ever-evolving fight against cancer, a new army has arisen – tumor-infiltrating lymphocyte (TIL) therapy. This audacious approach harnesses the body's own immune cells, those that have already braved the treacherous tumor microenvironment and engaged the malignant foe, extracting them from the very heart of the battle and fortifying their ranks for a renewed offensive.

The saga of TIL therapy unfolds as a tale of unwavering determination and ingenuity. First, a biopsy of the tumor is performed, a daring surgical strike to retrieve a sample of the adversary's stronghold. From this bounty, the intrepid researchers isolate the tumor-infiltrating lymphocytes, those valiant T-cells that have already infiltrated the enemy.

In the laboratory, these killer cells undergo proliferation, their numbers swelling through the power of cytokines, which fuels their exponential growth. Once their ranks have swelled to formidable proportions, they are reinfused into the patient's body; their mission is reignited with renewed vigor against the malignant adversaries.

In a landmark moment, the FDA approved Lifileucel, a TIL therapy developed by Iovance Biotherapeutics, for treating advanced melanoma. This momentous decision, born from data from clinical trials that unveiled significant clinical benefits in patients with metastatic melanoma, set a precedent for future therapies in this emerging weapon.

As the chronicles of TIL therapy continue to unfold, each chapter etched in the annals of scientific exploration stands as a beacon of hope for patients grappling with advanced malignancies, offering a personalized treatment option where others have faltered. The indomitable spirit that has propelled this quest burns ever brighter, illuminating the path toward a future where the scourge of cancer is defeated, one valiant stride at a time.

Tumor Vaccines

Tumor vaccines have proved to be another promising strategy for cancer immunotherapy, as they activate the body's immune system. Among the various types of tumor vaccines, dendritic cell (DC) vaccines, mRNA vaccines, and neoantigen vaccines have attracted much interest because they stimulate the precise anti-tumor immune response.

DC Vaccines: DC vaccines require cultures of dendritic cells, antigen-presenting cells recognized to play a central role in immunization and regulation of such processes. When removed from the patient's body, these cells are exposed to tumor antigens and subsequently reinfused back into the patient to generate a specific immune response against the tumors. The investigations involving DC vaccines have indicated their capacity to stimulate anti-tumor T cell responses in preclinical and clinical trials. However, the efficacy of DC vaccines is so far disappointing in the clinic for cancer treatment.

mRNA Vaccines: mRNA vaccines are one of the advanced techniques in cancer immunotherapy as they use synthetic mRNA molecules that construct antigens related to tumors to provoke a response from the immune system. These vaccines are meant to introduce tumor-specific antigens directly into host cells so that they are translated into proteins, thus stimulating the antigen-presenting cells and generating anti-tumor immunity. The advantages of mRNA vaccines are the exceptional speed of development, changes in which tumor-specific antigens should be focused, and even individual treatment. More recently, mRNA COVID-19 vaccines have proven effective and have boosted the exploration of mRNA vaccines in cancer immunotherapy. However, there remain concerns about the efficacy of mRNA vaccines against cancer

Neoantigen Vaccines: Neoantigen vaccines are developed by identifying tumor-specific mutations known as neoantigens due to changes in the cancer cell genome. These vaccines are developed from neoantigens found in each patient's tumor and do not target a person's normal cells but specific cancerous cells, making them unique to the patient. Neoantigen vaccines targeting cancer cells shall encourage the generation of T cells with the potential of identifying and killing cancer cells with these neoantigens without affecting normal cells. Recent achievements in the high-throughput sequencing and optimization of bioinformatics tools enable the discovery and rank of neoantigens for the development of vaccines. Neoantigen vaccines have been tested in several clinical trials for cancer, and the results obtained are pretty positive, such as tumor regression and a rise in the overall survival time in some patients. Nevertheless, difficulties like neoantigen variability, immune escape, and the reality of advanced bioprocessing are to be addressed.

Oncolytic Virus-Mediated Tumor Vaccines: These novel vaccines rely on oncolytic viruses (OV), which are viruses that can selectively replicate in and kill cancer cells. OVs are introduced into the body to attack tumor cells without affecting normal cells. The first is virally mediated cell lysis, in which the virus infects the tumor cells and multiplies within them before destroying them. This lysis liberates the tumor antigens in a rather immunogenic environment that notifies the immune system of the existence of cancer. Moreover, some OVs produce therapeutic genes that activate an immune response, increase viral replication, or change cancer's microenvironment, allowing immune cells to penetrate and eliminate cancer cells.

The principal advantage of using OVs as tumor vaccines lies in their dual action: it is based on direct oncolysis of the tumor and stimulation of systemic immune response against the tumor mass. Substantial progress has been achieved, and some OVs have been developed and approved by the FDA for treating melanoma and head and neck cancer, including T-VEC, Oncorine, and Pelareorep. Scientists are also working on developing combination therapies using OVs with other types of immunotherapies, like checkpoint inhibitors, with the hope of boosting the effectiveness of the treatments and overcoming issues of resistance to the exclusive treatments. Ongoing clinical trials are focused on determining the side effects profile, the doses of the combined treatments, and ultimate therapeutic outcomes.

Nevertheless, several issues remain in applying oncolytic virus-mediated tumor vaccines in clinics. One challenge is transporting the virus to the tumor cells, as the body's immune system quickly disposes of it before it can reach the tumor cells. This is where new insights in viral engineering and delivery must significantly improve the situation.

Over the last three decades, my research team has developed a range of innovative tumor vaccines leveraging dendritic cells, mRNA, and oncolytic virus technologies. Our preclinical studies, which showed promising results, paved the way for several clinical trials. These trials confirmed the vaccines' ability to elicit anti-tumor immune responses and sometimes prolong life. Despite these successes, the vaccines have not yet been able to eradicate tumors or maintain prolonged anti-tumor efficacy in cancer patients.

Tumor vaccines represent a promising frontier in cancer immunotherapy, offering the potential for precise and durable anti-tumor immune responses. However, continued development is needed to fully harness the immune system's power to kill cancer cells with sufficient efficacy.

Personalized Precision Therapy

Personalized or precision cancer therapy is an innovative approach to cancer treatment that tailors medical care to the specific genetic profile of a patient's tumor. This approach involves analyzing the genetic mutations and alterations in a patient's cancer cells to create a "tumor profile." Based on this genetic profile, doctors can select therapies that specifically target the unique characteristics of the patient's cancer, potentially leading to more effective treatments with fewer side effects compared to traditional one-size-fits-all approaches.

The implementation of precision medicine in cancer care relies heavily on advanced technologies such as next-generation DNA sequencing and large-scale data analysis. These tools allow clinicians to identify key genetic changes, biomarkers, and other molecular features that guide treatment decisions. Precision medicine is currently being used for several cancer types, including colorectal, breast, lung, and certain types of leukemia and lymphoma. In these cases, tumors are typically tested for specific gene or protein changes at diagnosis or during treatment to inform therapeutic choices.

While precision medicine has shown great promise in certain cancers, it is still an evolving field with ongoing research to expand its application to more cancer types. Challenges include the complexity of tumor biology, the development of drug resistance, and the need for more comprehensive genetic testing. Despite these hurdles, precision cancer therapy represents a significant advancement in oncology, offering the potential for more targeted and effective treatments. As research progresses, the hope is that treatments will be increasingly customized to the specific gene and protein changes in each patient's cancer, ultimately improving outcomes and quality of life for cancer patients.

Successful Treatment for Hematologic and Some Solid malignancies

Recent scientific breakthroughs in immunotherapy, targeted therapies, and personalized medicine have successfully treated certain types of cancer.

Melanoma. Once a grim diagnosis, metastatic melanoma has seen a dramatic transformation with the advent of immunotherapy and targeted treatments. Checkpoint inhibitors such as pembrolizumab and nivolumab have harnessed the body's immune system to fight the disease, achieving a 33% overall response rate and a five-year survival rate of approximately 34% in previously incurable cases. The combination of BRAF and MEK inhibitors, like dabrafenib and trametinib, has shown an impressive 70% response rate and nearly 28% five-year survival in BRAF-mutant metastatic melanoma. Today, early detection and advanced treatments have significantly improved outcomes, with the American Cancer Society reporting a 92% five-year survival rate across all melanoma stages. Even in the most severe metastatic cases, the five-year survival rate has risen to 27%, offering a glimmer of hope.

A subset of colon cancer. In colon cancer, particularly for tumors with specific genetic profiles, these innovative approaches have shown remarkable results. Microsatellite Instability-High (MSI-H) tumors, accounting for about 15% of colon cancers, have significantly responded to immunotherapy drugs called checkpoint inhibitors, improving outcomes and survival rates. Additionally, targeted therapies combining BRAF inhibitors with other agents have shown promising results in clinical trials for patients with BRAF V600E mutated tumors, a subset traditionally associated with poor prognosis.

Hematopoietic malignancies. Hematopoietic malignancies, including leukemias and lymphomas, have seen some of the most dramatic improvements in treatment outcomes. Targeted therapies have revolutionized treatment for various blood cancers. For instance, rituximab, an anti-CD20 antibody, has significantly improved outcomes for many B-cell lymphomas, with the addition of rituximab to standard chemotherapy improving 5-year survival rates in diffuse large B-cell lymphoma from about

50% to 70-80%. In chronic lymphocytic leukemia, targeted therapies such as BTK and BCL-2 inhibitors have offered high response rates and improved patient survival.

CAR T-cell therapy has emerged as a groundbreaking treatment for certain hematopoietic malignancies. CAR T-cell therapy has shown remarkable success in acute lymphoblastic leukemia, with complete remission rates of 80-90% reported in clinical trials. Similarly, for relapsed or refractory B cell lymphoma, CAR T-cell therapy has demonstrated promising results with overall response rates of 50-80% in various studies.

These successes highlight the potential of personalized, precision medicine approaches in cancer treatment, significantly improving outcomes for many patients by tailoring treatments to their tumors' specific genetic or molecular characteristics.

Dismal Reality: Metastatic Cancer Remains Largely Incurable

Despite these advances, the dismal reality is that metastatic cancer remains an unconquered frontier. Despite the countless billions invested in research and the technological marvels harnessed in this war, the majority of patients diagnosed with late-stage, widespread disease ultimately succumb to its onslaught. Current treatments often prove futile once cancer has spread, highlighting the limitations in our arsenal.

Chemotherapies, radiation, and targeted therapies may initially cause tumors to retreat, only for them to reemerge in new sites with renewed ferocity. We may strike them down, but they are reborn, more defiant and diverse than before. This relentless cycle of treatment, remission and relapse often ends in the same way for most—a losing battle against an implacable foe.

Even our most advanced immunotherapies, hailed as game-changers capable of rallying the body's defenses, struggle to overcome cancer's boundless immune evasion and resistance capacity. Temporary remissions offer hope but rarely deliver a lasting cure. The metastatic disease persists, adapting and outmaneuvering each new treatment we deploy. Recent data illustrate the difficulty of treating advanced-stage cancer; for example, the 5-year survival rate is less than 1% for patients with stage 4B non-small cell lung cancer, even with a formidable arsenal of drugs.

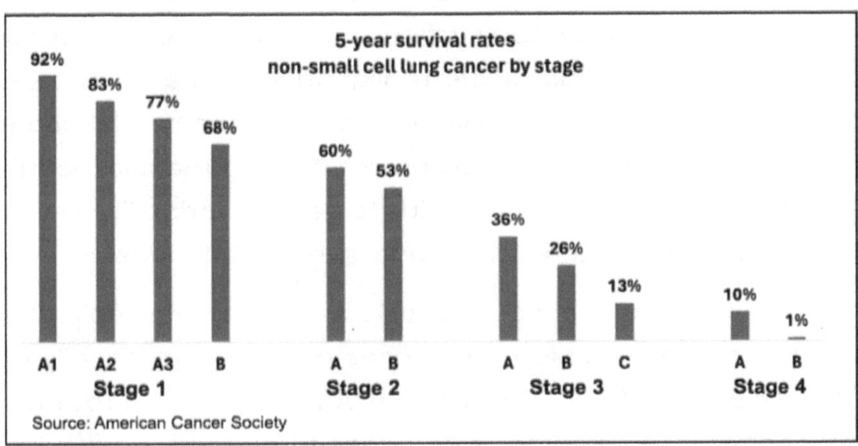

For every remission that defies the odds, there are legions of other patients for whom medicine's front line proves hopelessly outmatched against cancer's vicious spread. Victory remains elusive, a sobering reminder of how formidable an adversary we face in this endless war.

Why is Metastatic Cancer Treatment Still So Ineffective?

Cancer is a master of deception, a shape-shifting adversary that refuses to be confined by the rules we attempt to impose. At its core lies an unsettling heterogeneity — tumors that appear identical on the surface can harbor staggering genetic diversity within. This complexity is the enemy's greatest strength, allowing it to adapt and evolve with insidious ingenuity. Here are some significant reasons for the difficulty of eradicating metastatic cancer.

Metastatic Tumor Complexity and Resilience. In the chronicles of medical research, few challenges are as daunting as finding a cure for metastatic cancer. Despite significant scientific advancements, this elusive adversary remains a mystery, constantly adapting and resisting even the most determined efforts to defeat it.

The Mutational Maelstrom. Metabolic flux, a host, is encased in the cell's shield to the extent that the genetic diversity heralds metastatic cancer. Cancers are characterized by presumptuous genomic heterogeneity; each tumor harbors numerous mutations that form the genotype of the malignancy. Some of these are determinants of the progression of the malignancy, while others are innocent bystanders. Hence, even if the treatment is meant to be very specific, it may not work due to genetic variability, which is a stumbling block in achieving a one-size-fits-all model.

Adding another layer of complexity, tumors are not simple tissue knots but complexes. Many subclones are often genetically and phenotypically different from each other—that is, intratumoral heterogeneity. This internal heterogeneity creates a difficulty in that therapies that exterminate one subclone may not affect other subclones, and thus, the disease may return. The complexity is realized mainly in situations with intertumoral heterogeneity. Metastases, those secondary growths that disseminate the illness, bear various genetic characteristics that differ from their original companion tumors due to the new sites' conditions.

The Specter of Adaptation--Resistance and Escape Mutations. Metastatic cancer is not only a diverse entity but a robust and tenacious foe because of its capacity to adapt and read the attempts at its destruction. Targeted therapies or chemotherapy can activate the other signaling pathways or alter the phenotype of the malignant cells, and thus, the treatment methods become ineffective.

This adaptive resistance is demonstrated when fighting chronic myeloid leukemia, also known as CML. As to molecular targeted agents, tyrosine kinase inhibitors of BCR-ABL, such as imatinib, have yielded only BCR-ABL gene mutations requiring second and third generations.

However, these reinforcements are not foolproof, as cancer wields a particularly insidious weapon: Among escape mutations, there are three types, which are Rates of phenotypic and genotypic change, Fitness, and macro-evolution. Such genetic mutations within the target gene or other related pathways endow the tumors with resistance to the therapies intended to eliminate them. An example in lung cancer is the T790M resistance mutation that has rendered first-generation EGFR inhibitors ineffective, and there has been research to establish counteraction methods.

The Tumor Microenvironment. In addition to genetic muscle, metastatic cancer fights the rapidly shifting character of the tumor microenvironment, a battleground of stromal cells, immune cells, blood vessels, and extracellular matrix. This environment can either constitute a limitation that thwarts the development of the malignancy and its resistance to therapy or a suitable environment that promotes it. Hypoxic areas of tumors are remote to the effects of radiotherapy and chemotherapy. Moreover, metastatic tumors abuse the host immunity by recruiting Regulatory T cells and Myeloid-derived suppressor cells, which hinder immunity. They also produce immune checkpoint molecules such as PD-L1 and cover themselves to evade immune system destruction.

Studying these mechanisms will allow for a better understanding of how best to fight metastatic cancer, sustainably enhancing the chances of patients' survival.

Undying Dream of Finding a Cure
In the intricate and resilient journey against metastatic cancer, finding a cure still faces formidable challenges. This quest is complicated by the disease's unique genetic mutations, the

adaptability of cancer cells, and the emergence of escape mutations that defy even the most tailored treatments.

Yet, amidst these daunting hurdles, the relentless spirit of scientific exploration shines brighter than ever. Ongoing research into the molecular foundations of cancer, coupled with advanced therapies and personalized medicine, offers a beacon of hope to penetrate the defenses of this relentless enemy.

In this monumental struggle, each advance and every hard-fought victory bring us closer to our ultimate goal: a future where metastatic cancer is obliterated. This unwavering aspiration fuels our collective resolve, driving us forward despite overwhelming odds.

This is our undying dream: one day, we will find a cure for advanced cancer!

The Barrier of Non-Modifiable Risk Factors in Prevention

CHAPTER THREE

"An ounce of prevention is worth a pound of cure."
Benjamin Franklin

What is the key barrier to effective cancer prevention?

Our journey to conquer cancer has been marked by significant advancements in cancer treatment. Despite these achievements, metastatic cancer remains largely incurable, with an overall five-year survival rate of < 20% for most cancer types. This stark statistic highlights the limitations of treatments, which often provide only marginal therapeutic benefits or palliative care for patients with advanced disease.

Having dedicated over three decades to developing cutting-edge cancer treatments, I am both disheartened and motivated by this harsh reality. While we have made notable progress, the relentless march of this insidious disease continues to claim millions of lives, prompting a critical reflection on our strategies—are we genuinely targeting the most effective fronts?

With no cure for advanced cancer on the horizon, this bleak reality forces us to shift our focus from seeking a cure to revisiting an age-old strategy—prevention, aiming to defeat the disease at its very inception.

This chapter will showcase the advances and successes in cancer prevention by reducing modifiable risk factors.

Yet, the incidence of cancer continues to rise both in the US and worldwide despite significant strides in preventive practices. This chapter will subsequently delve into the challenges of cancer prevention due to non-modifiable or non-preventable risk factors like aging, highlighting the need for early detection as a crucial secondary prevention measure.

Risk Factors of Cancer

Cancer is a master of deception and unpredictability, capable of striking at nearly any organ or tissue—be it the lung, colon, breast, skin, bones, or even delicate nerve tissue. This insidious disease, encompassing a group of maladies characterized by the uncontrolled growth and spread of malignant cells, has waged an unrelenting war against the fortresses of our bodies.

Cancer's true menace lies in its ability to metastasize, spreading its malignant reach throughout the body by infiltrating the blood and lymphatic systems. It is a foe that knows no boundaries, ever-adapting, ever-evolving, and ever-seeking new footholds from which to wage its relentless assault.

At the heart of cancer's onslaught lies a betrayal of the most fundamental principles of life itself—the corruption of the very genetic code that governs cellular behavior. It is a disease born of multiple DNA mutations, a sinister symphony of genetic errors that unleashes the growth of abnormal cells, unbound by the constraints that once kept them in check.

In this epic struggle, however, knowledge is power. By comprehending the roots and risk factors that fuel cancer, we can arm ourselves with the tools necessary to safeguard our health and thwart the onset of this formidable foe.

These risk factors, the harbingers of cancer's advance and invasion, come in many forms. Some are modifiable, born of our choices and lifestyles—habits and behaviors that can be reshaped and reformed. Others are non-modifiable, the immutable forces of nature that we cannot alter but must learn to navigate with wisdom and vigilance.

Understanding these risk factors—distinguishing the modifiable from the immutable—enables us to chart a course for cancer prevention. This proactive stance begins not in operating theaters or laboratories but in our daily choices, how we nourish our bodies, and how we fortify our defenses against this relentless adversary.

Non-Modifiable Risk Factors

Non-modifiable risk factors are those beyond our control, such as age, genetics, gender, and race/ethnicity. These factors are immutable in their nature.

Age is the most significant risk factor for cancer. The National Cancer Institute (NCI) reports that the median age of cancer diagnosis is 66 years. Genetic mutations can accumulate in our cells as we age, increasing cancer risk over time.

Genetics refers to the inherited traits passed down from our parents. Certain germline mutations, like BRCA1 and BRCA2, significantly raise the risk of developing cancers such as breast and ovarian cancer. However, it's crucial to note that only 5-10% of all cancers are attributed to hereditary genetic mutations.

Gender, encompassing the biological differences between males and females, influences cancer risk. For example, prostate cancer is prevalent among men, while breast cancer predominantly affects women. Hormonal imbalances play a critical role in these disparities, highlighting the intricate relationship between biology and disease. Additionally, cancer rates can vary across racial and ethnic groups due to genetic and environmental factors.

While non-modifiable or non-preventable factors cannot be changed, awareness of these risks is vital for tailoring cancer screening and prevention strategies.

Modifiable Risk Factors

In the landscape of risk factors, some are within our control and shaped by our actions and choices. These modifiable factors include behaviors and lifestyle choices such as tobacco and alcohol use, obesity, viral infections, and environmental exposures. By addressing these modifiable risk factors, individuals can substantially lower their risk of developing cancer.

- Cigarette Smoking and Secondhand Smoke: Active smoking, as well as passive smoking, is one of the significant risks for several types of cancer, such as lung cancer, throat cancer, and mouth cancer. Cigarette smoking is widely known to cause cancer, and statistics show that it contributes to as much as 22% of global cancer fatalities. Its chemicals act in ways that mutate the cell, causing it to become dangerous cancer cells.

- Excess Body Weight: Obesity escalates the probability of developing cancers of the breast, colon, and kidney, among others. Obesity is linked to 14% of males and 20% of female's cancer deaths since it interferes with hormonal homeostasis and triggers chronic inflammations that assist malignant cell growth. High circulating levels of insulin and growth factors that are present in overweight persons fuel cancer growth.

- Alcohol Consumption: Consumption of alcohol increases the chances of developing certain types of cancer, for instance, breast, liver, and esophageal cancer.

- Red and Processed Meat: Red and processed meats are known cancer hazards that increase the chances of developing cancer, such as colon cancer.

- Low Intake of Fruits, Vegetables, Dietary Fiber, and Calcium: Lack of such components makes one vulnerable to colon cancer as such substances as fruits, vegetables, and fiber possess protective characteristics.

- Physical Inactivity: Lack of exercise may increase the chances of acquiring various types of cancer, including breast and colon cancer.

- Exposure to carcinogens. Most skin cancers result from ultraviolet (UV) radiation from sunshine or tanning equipment. The environment plays a key role in the occurrence of many cases of cancer among individuals. Contamination by dangerous chemicals and radiation can cause changes or mutations in the DNA and create cancer cells. For example, fibers found in asbestos can lead to lung cancer. It is crucial to minimize interaction with various carcinogens as much as possible and wear sun creams and gear when faced with possibly risky regions.

- Cancer-Associated Infections: Hepatitis B and C viruses are other known causes of liver cancer. Human Papillomavirus (HPV) is known to cause the majority of cervical cancer cases and is related to genital and head and neck cancers. Helicobacter pylori cause stomach cancer.

Cancer Prevention by Reducing Modifiable Risk Factors

In the battle against cancer, our daily choices serve as powerful defenses. While some risk factors, like age, are beyond our control, many others are within our reach to mitigate.

By avoiding tobacco, we eliminate a major source of carcinogens found in cigarettes and chewing tobacco. Our dietary habits also play a crucial role, either promoting cancer growth with sugary, fatty, processed foods or combating it with wholesome, plant-based options.

Regular exercise strengthens our body's defenses against cancer, while a sedentary lifestyle leaves us vulnerable. Limiting alcohol consumption, practicing safe sex, and adhering to vaccination schedules add additional layers of protection.

The sun's ultraviolet rays present a covert threat, damaging DNA with each unprotected exposure. Wearing protective clothing and using sunscreen diligently serve as our shield against this invisible enemy.

Ultimately, our daily choices hold significant sway over our cancer risk. While complete prevention remains elusive, addressing these modifiable risks establishes a formidable first line of defense against cancer and other diseases. Common recommendations for cancer prevention by reducing modifiable risk factors are listed in the accompanying table.

In summary, though complete prevention remains beyond our grasp, mitigating modifiable risk factors as preventive measures has reduced cancer incidence.

Common Recommendations for Cancer Prevention

Recommendation	Description
Avoid Tobacco	Refrain from smoking or using tobacco products.
Eat a Healthy Diet	Consume a diet rich in fruits, vegetables, whole grains, and lean proteins; limit processed and red meats.
Maintain a Healthy Weight	Keep a healthy body weight through a balanced diet and regular exercise.
Be Physically Active	Engage in regular physical activity, aiming for at least 150 minutes of moderate exercise per week.
Limit Alcohol Consumption	If you drink alcohol, do so in moderation: up to one drink per day for women and two for men.
Protect Yourself from the Sun	Use sunscreen, wear protective clothing, and avoid tanning beds.
Get Vaccinated	Get vaccines for viruses like HPV and Hepatitis B, which can increase cancer risk.
Avoid Risky Behaviors	Practice safe sex and avoid sharing needles to reduce the risk of infections that can lead to cancer.
Get Regular Medical Care	Attend regular check-ups and cancer screenings as recommended by your healthcare provider.
Reduce Exposure to Environmental Toxins	Minimize exposure to known carcinogens, such as asbestos, radon, and certain chemicals.
Stay Informed	Keep updated on new research and guidelines for cancer prevention.

Gloomy Reality: The Rising Incidence of Cancer

Despite the progress in cancer prevention, the specter of this disease continues to loom large. The global burden of cancer is projected to grow by a staggering 77% by 2050, reaching 35.4 million new cases annually. In the United States alone, new cancer cases rose from 1.9 million in 2022 to over 2 million in 2023, with an estimated 2,001,140 new cases anticipated in 2024 (NCI Cancer Statistics). A confluence of formidable factors drives this alarming surge.

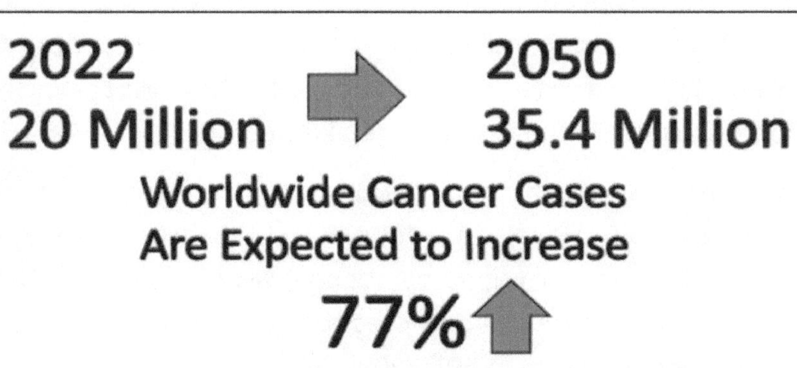

At the forefront is the relentless march of time and the demographic shift towards older populations. Advances in healthcare and living conditions have extended life expectancies worldwide, with the number of people over 60 expected to reach 2.1 billion by 2050 (WHO, 2022). In the United States, the proportion of individuals aged 65 and older is set to rise from 16% in 2019 to a staggering 23% by 2060 (US Census Bureau, 2020).

Aging, an insidious ally of cancer, leads to the accumulation of genetic mutations and the weakening of immune defenses, increasing the likelihood of malignancy. It is a sobering reality that 60% of all cancer cases and 70% of cancer deaths occur in those aged 65 and older, with breast, prostate, colorectal, and lung cancers being the most prevalent. Cancers are caused by mutations that may be inherited, induced by environmental carcinogens, or result from random DNA replication errors. There is a strong correlation between cancer incidence and normal stem cell divisions, regardless of the environment. Random mutations may account for two-thirds of the mutations in human cancers (*Science* 2017). These findings align with epidemiological estimates that environmental changes can only prevent a fraction of cancers.

The incidence rates for cancer steadily increase with age, from fewer than 25 cases per 100,000 people in those under 20, to about 350 per 100,000 among individuals aged 45–49, and to more than 1,000 per 100,000 in those aged 60 and older. The cancer incidence rate increases 40-fold between ages 20 and 60.

Adding to the peril of an aging population is the relentless obesity epidemic. By 2016, 1.9 billion adults worldwide were overweight, with over 650 million classified as obese (WHO, 2022). In the United States, the crisis has reached unprecedented levels, with over 42% of adults deemed obese in 2017-2018.

Obesity, a catalyst for chronic inflammation, insulin resistance, and hormonal imbalances, has proven to be a potent ally in cancer's arsenal. Excess body weight has been implicated in cancers such as breast, colorectal, endometrial, kidney, liver, pancreatic, and esophageal, contributing to an estimated 3.9% of all cancers globally in 2012. In this ever-evolving battleground, the combined onslaught of aging populations, rising obesity rates, and increasing physical inactivity presents a formidable challenge for cancer prevention.

To sum up, the success of prevention lights a path beckoning us to make even greater efforts to mitigate modifiable cancer risk factors. However, even the best prevention efforts still fall short of their true mark, as the insurmountable obstacle of the biggest risk factor—aging—looms large, threatening the progress of cancer prevention.

The obstacle of non-modifiable risk factors underscores the importance of early detection as a secondary cancer prevention measure, aiming to prevent deaths from cancers caused by unavoidable random mutations that accumulate with aging, which will be explored in the next chapter.

Huge Gaps in Early Detection

"Early detection is crucial. It can mean the difference between life and death. Don't wait, get screened today."
Sheryl Crow

What are the major obstacles to effective cancer screening and early detection?

While prevention plays a substantial role in reducing cancer risk, it cannot overcome the looming challenge of aging, a non-preventable risk factor. Thus, early detection, as a form of secondary prevention, is imperative in order to defeat this formidable disease.

The importance of early detection in cancer treatment cannot be overstated. Cancers detected at early, localized stages are often curable without the need for aggressive, comprehensive therapies. For instance, early-stage breast cancer has a >90% five-year survival rate. Moreover, early detection substantially lowers healthcare costs by reducing the need for invasive, prolonged, and comprehensive treatments, which are largely ineffective, economically burdensome, and detrimental to patients' overall quality of life.

This chapter will review the successes of current cancer screening and early detection for several types of cancer using single-site or single-organ screening tests to save lives.

This chapter will then discuss significant gaps in current cancer screening tests since the majority of all cancer deaths result from cancers, including deadly pancreatic, ovarian, liver, kidney, bone, and brain cancers, without recommended screening tests. Beyond better implementation of current single-site screening tests, advancing innovative early detection technologies is crucial to fill the significant gaps in cancer early detection.

Current Single-Site Cancer Screening Tests

Cancer Screening Tests Currently Recommended by USPSTF for Women and Men

Cancer Screening Tests for Women

Cancer Type	Screening Test	Population	Frequency
Breast Cancer	Mammography	Women aged 50 to 74	Every 2 years
Cervical Cancer	Pap smear (Pap test) and/or HPV testing	Women aged 21 to 65	Pap test every 3 years; HPV test every 5 years (or combined every 5 years for women aged 30 to 65)
Colorectal Cancer	Colonoscopy, Sigmoidoscopy, FIT, FOBT	Adults aged 45 to 75	Varies by test (1–10 years)
Lung Cancer	Low-dose computed tomography (LDCT)	Adults aged 50 to 80 with a 20 pack-year smoking history, current smokers or those who have quit within the past 15 years	Annually

Cancer Screening Tests for Men

Cancer Type	Screening Test	Population	Frequency
Colorectal Cancer	Colonoscopy, Sigmoidoscopy, FIT, FOBT	Adults aged 45 to 75	Varies by test (1–10 years)
Lung Cancer	Low-dose computed tomography (LDCT)	Adults aged 50 to 80 with a 20 pack-year smoking history, current smokers or those who have quit within the past 15 years	Annually
Prostate Cancer	Prostate-specific antigen (PSA) test	Men aged 55 to 69	Individual decision

Early-stage cancers are often curable due to the confinement to their site of origin, making complete surgical removal feasible. The prospect of achieving a cure is most promising at this pivotal moment. Rigorous screening for breast, cervical, colorectal, and other cancers allows us to strike before the disease can spread, shifting the balance in our favor.

Presently, the US Preventive Services Task Force (USPSTF) endorses single-site cancer screening tests for breast, colorectal, cervical, and lung cancer for individuals at risk, which will be summarized in the table and described below.

Mammography for Breast Cancer Screening

Mammography serves as a fundamental tool in the detection and screening of breast cancer. This non-invasive imaging technique utilizes low-dose X-rays to identify signs of breast cancer in asymptomatic women.

Gaining traction in the late 1950s and early 1960s, mammography achieved widespread acceptance by the 1970s, bolstered by studies highlighting its effectiveness in the early detection of breast cancer. The introduction of digital breast tomosynthesis, or 3D mammography, in the early 21st century enhanced this process by providing a layered view of the breast, which helps improve cancer detection by minimizing tissue overlap that can obscure tumors.

Screening guidelines have evolved over the years. The American Cancer Society recommends annual mammograms for women aged 45 to 54 and biennial or yearly screenings for those aged 55 and older, tailored to individual preferences and health histories. However, recommendations can differ among organizations, considering personal risk and breast density factors.

Extensive research has shown that regular mammography screenings can detect breast cancers at earlier stages, leading to better treatment outcomes and lower mortality rates. A meta-analysis of randomized trials demonstrated that mammography screening significantly reduces breast cancer mortality, particularly among women aged 50 to 69.

Despite its advantages, mammography screening has sparked discussions regarding issues such as overdiagnosis and false positives. Overdiagnosis refers to detecting cancers that would not have led to harm, resulting in unnecessary treatments. False positives—instances where cancer is erroneously indicated—can cause significant anxiety and necessitate further testing. Critics advocate for personalized screening strategies to balance the benefits of early detection with the risks associated with overdiagnosis and false positives.

Pap Smear and HPV Testing for Cervical Cancer Screening

The Pap smear test, developed by Dr. George Papanicolaou in the early 20th century, involves the collection of cervical cells, which are then examined under a microscope for abnormalities. This groundbreaking method has played a crucial role in significantly reducing both the incidence and mortality rates of cervical cancer.

When paired with HPV testing, the effectiveness of cervical cancer screening is further enhanced. HPV testing identifies high-risk strains of the virus that cause cervical cancer. Combining both tests improves the detection of precancerous lesions, offering better detection than the Pap smear alone. Several HPV tests have received FDA approval as primary screening tools or for co-testing alongside the Pap smear, meeting established performance standards for detecting HPV infections and cervical abnormalities.

Current guidelines for cervical cancer screening recommend the inclusion of both Pap smear and HPV testing. The American Cancer Society advises that screening begins at age 25, recommending primary HPV testing every five years. Alternatively, women aged 25 to 65 may opt for co-testing every five years or

Pap smears alone every three years, reflecting advancements in detection methods and extended screening intervals. When combined with regular screening, vaccination significantly lowers the incidence of cervical cancer.

Colonoscopy for Colorectal Cancer Screening

Colonoscopy plays a vital role in the fight against colorectal cancer, which is the third most prevalent cancer in the United States. By facilitating early detection and the removal of precancerous polyps, this procedure significantly lowers the risk of developing cancer. During a colonoscopy, a gastroenterologist utilizes a flexible tube fitted with a camera to examine the rectum and colon, enabling the visualization and extraction of abnormal tissues. Research has demonstrated its effectiveness in identifying early-stage colorectal cancer and preventing the progression of polyps.

The FDA regulates the devices employed in colonoscopies, while organizations like the USPSTF and the American Cancer Society provide screening guidelines. Current recommendations suggest initiating screening at age 50; however, due to increasing colorectal cancer rates among younger individuals, the American Cancer Society now recommends beginning screenings at age 45 for those at average risk.

Early detection through colonoscopy greatly enhances survival rates by identifying cancer at curable stages. Additionally, the removal of precancerous polyps serves to prevent the development of cancer, highlighting the procedure's dual role in both prevention and diagnosis. Regular screenings significantly decrease colorectal cancer mortality.

Low-dose Chest CT for Lung Cancer Screening

In the battle against cancer, few adversaries rival the threat of lung cancer. This insidious disease often goes undetected until it reaches advanced stages, severely limiting treatment options and leading to dismal outcomes. However, a new screening tool has emerged: the low-dose computed tomography (LDCT) scan.

Traditional methods for detecting lung cancer, such as chest X-rays and sputum cytology, have consistently underperformed in identifying the disease in its early, treatable stages. Their limited sensitivity frequently results in late diagnoses. In contrast, LDCT excels at spotting even the tiniest nodules, which are early indicators of malignancy.

The National Lung Screening Trial (NLST) marked a pivotal moment in lung cancer detection, demonstrating LDCT's capabilities. The study revealed a 20% reduction in lung cancer mortality compared to chest X-rays. When lung cancer is identified at an early stage, the five-year survival rate can soar to an impressive 56%, compared to a mere 5% for advanced-stage disease. This critical window is where LDCT shines, offering a beacon of hope and a chance to change the outcome.

While the initial cost of LDCT screening may appear steep, the long-term savings from reduced treatment expenses for early-stage cancers make it a financially sound strategy. Research published in The *New England Journal of Medicine* confirms LDCT's cost-effectiveness.

Leading health organizations, including the USPSTF and the American Cancer Society, endorse LDCT screening, recommending it for high-risk individuals—specifically, those aged 50 to 80 with a 20-pack-year smoking history, as well as current or recent smokers.

Despite LDCT's numerous successes, potential risks persist. Although the radiation dose is lower than that of standard CT scans, annual screenings raise concerns about radiation-induced malignancies. Additionally, the high rate of false positives—96% in the NLST trial—necessitates further imaging and invasive procedures to eliminate non-cancerous findings. Nevertheless, ongoing research and technological advancements hold promise for refining LDCT screening. Improved risk stratification and the integration of artificial intelligence aim to reduce false positives and optimize screening intervals.

PSA Test for Prostate Cancer Screening

The Prostate-Specific Antigen (PSA) test is a blood test for prostate cancer screening and has been a fundamental aspect of men's health for decades. This test measures the levels of PSA, a protein produced by both cancerous and noncancerous prostate tissues.

The PSA test identifies elevated PSA levels, which may indicate early-stage prostate cancer or benign conditions like prostatitis or benign prostatic hyperplasia (BPH). It complicates the test's specificity for detecting cancer. Despite this challenge, the PSA test remains an invaluable tool for the early detection of prostate cancer, often identifying the disease before symptoms arise.

The FDA's approval of the PSA test in the early 1990s marked an advance in prostate cancer screening. Since then, its use has become widespread, though not without controversy. Critics contend that the PSA test can result in overdiagnosis and overtreatment of prostate cancers that may never develop into clinically significant issues. This situation highlights the risks associated with treatment, which can include side effects such as incontinence and erectile dysfunction.

In light of these concerns, screening guidelines have evolved. The USPSTF recommends that men aged 55 to 69 discuss PSA screening with their healthcare providers, weighing personal values against the benefits and risks of the test. For men over 70, routine PSA screening is generally discouraged.

Advances in Molecular Tests for Cancer Screening

Molecular testing is transforming oncology and paving the way for personalized cancer screening and care. By analyzing genetic mutations, biomarkers, and gene expressions, these tests offer vital insights into cancer risk, early detection, and customized treatment approaches.

At the core of molecular testing lies the understanding of cancer's genetic foundations. By deciphering DNA alterations that influence cellular behavior, these tests can identify the presence of cancer before symptoms manifest. Molecular tests for cancer screening evaluate biological markers within the genome and proteome— such as DNA, RNA, proteins, and metabolites—to assess an individual's cancer risk, detect the presence of cancer, or predict the disease's progression. For cancers such as lung, colorectal, and breast cancer, molecular testing is increasingly essential for early diagnosis and tailored treatment plans.

Recent advancements in molecular screening tests for cancer detection, approved by the FDA in 2024, have significantly enhanced early cancer diagnosis and management. Notable innovations include non-invasive stool RNA tests for colorectal cancer and state-of-the-art blood tests for colorectal neoplasia. The FDA has approved ColoSense, a multitarget stool RNA test for colorectal cancer screening. This non-invasive test analyzes stool samples for RNA markers linked to colorectal cancer and advanced adenomas. In clinical trials, ColoSense demonstrated sensitivity and specificity comparable to existing molecular screening tests, offering a less invasive alternative to colonoscopy for cancer detection.

Another promising advancement is Guardant Health's Shield blood test, identifying circulating tumor DNA (ctDNA) related to colorectal cancer, which has been recommended for FDA approval for screening adults aged 45 and older at average risk in

2024. This test detects colorectal neoplasia by identifying genomic and epigenomic alterations in cfDNA from blood samples.

The FDA has also approved various tests for cancer screening across various cancer types. Among stool-based tests, Cologuard—a stool DNA test approved in 2014—detects mutations associated with colorectal cancer in adults aged 45 and older who are at average risk. Fecal Immunochemical Tests (FIT), which identify blood in stool indicative of colorectal cancer or precancerous polyps, have also been granted FDA approval. In the blood-based test category, CancerSEEK detects genetic mutations and protein biomarkers linked to multiple cancers, including pancreatic, ovarian, and liver cancers, and received FDA Breakthrough Device designation in 2019. In breast cancer, Oncotype DX analyzes the expression of 21 genes to predict recurrence risk and assess the benefits of chemotherapy. Meanwhile, MammaPrint evaluates 70 genes to classify metastatic risk as high or low, guiding decisions about adjuvant chemotherapy.

Other FDA-approved tests include EsoCheck, a non-invasive cell collection device cleared in 2019 to detect Barrett's esophagus—a precursor to esophageal cancer. The OVA1 blood test, approved in 2009, assesses ovarian cancer risk in women with an ovarian mass. The PCA3 urine test, approved in 2012, detects prostate cancer antigen 3 to determine the necessity of a prostate biopsy. ROMA, another blood test approved in 2011, predicts the risk of ovarian cancer in women presenting with a pelvic mass. The FDA continues to evaluate and approve new cancer screening tests to bolster early detection and prevention efforts across different cancer types. These new molecular screening tests signify a substantial advance in cancer detection, providing more sensitive, specific, and less invasive options for early diagnosis.

Significant Gaps in Early Detection

In the ongoing fight against cancer, knowledge is the most potent weapon—especially awareness of the importance of screening for asymptomatic, early detection. However, a new report from NORC at the University of Chicago reveals that current cancer screening efforts are awfully inadequate.

On December 14, 2022, researchers revealed a startling fact: **only 14% of cancers in the United States are detected through recommended screening tests**. The remaining 86% are discovered through other means—either when symptoms appear or during unrelated medical care. These cancers are typically identified at later stages, accounting for 70% of cancer-related deaths.

Currently, only four types of cancer—breast, cervical, colorectal, and lung—benefit from screening tests recommended by the United States Preventive Services Task Force (USPSTF). Yet these screenings account for just 29% of all cancer cases diagnosed in the US.

NORC's report reveals that 57% of all diagnosed cancers come from types without a recommended screening test. These cancers often emerge only when symptoms appear, typically in later stages where treatment is much more challenging. These undetected cancers represent 70% of all cancer-related deaths, emphasizing the urgent need for improved detection methods.

These findings call for renewed action in cancer screening. "Cancer treatments have vastly improved over the last few decades," notes Caroline Pearson, senior vice president at NORC. "But the health system's ability to screen for cancer, which is essential for early diagnosis and effective treatment, still has a long way to go." Her words highlight the urgent need for more screening and early detection options.

The Need for New Technologies for Systemic Early Detection Throughout the Whole Body

Current screening tests examine specific organs or tissues one at a time. However, this piecemeal strategy is akin to searching a sprawling city one block at a time, leaving ample opportunity for malignancies to go unnoticed in unexplored districts. The enormity of this challenge calls for a revolutionary approach—a sweeping, systemic detection system capable of surveying the entire body in a single test.

Just as a city might deploy a sophisticated surveillance network to monitor all neighborhoods simultaneously, researchers envision a groundbreaking systemic cancer screening test capable of detecting cancer throughout the whole body.

The miracle of life is carried out by cells dividing and replicating themselves through countless cycles. In this intricate dance, each cellular factory must meticulously copy the billions of coded instructions that govern its existence—the DNA within the nucleus. However, this process is not infallible. Errors can creep in, subtly corrupting the code with each division. While many of these mutations are harmless, some can cause the cell to lose its way, multiplying uncontrollably and ignoring the finely-tuned signals that regulate growth. This is how a normal cell can transform into a cancer cell—a dangerous imposter cloaked in similarity to its healthy counterparts.

The human body is a vast metropolis of cells, with innumerable neighborhoods of specialized tissues and vital organ districts working in concert. Disturbingly, any single proliferating cell in this microscopic city has the potential to turn traitorous if mutations accumulate. This betrayal can occur silently. When symptoms arise, the insidious invaders may have already established footholds and spread throughout the body's landscape. There are more than 200 types of cancer, based on where they start in the body, such as breast cancer or lung cancer.

Achieving this ambitious vision of systemic early detection of the whole body will undoubtedly require overcoming numerous scientific and technical challenges, but the potential rewards are immense. A reliable, all-encompassing cancer detection system could dramatically improve outcomes and save countless lives by facilitating timely interventions against this relentless disease. In the battle to defeat cancer, such a systemic early-detection weapon would significantly tip the odds in favor of human defenders. Advancing this scientific frontier may represent our only effective path to ultimate victory over cancer's relentless scourge.

In summary, early detection has proven to be the most effective means for curing cancers. Thus, defeating cancer hinges on systemic early detection rather than finding a cure!

The pressing need now is how to fill the significant gaps in cancer screening tests for most cancer types, which will be extensively explored in the following chapters.

PART II

The Hope

Breakthrough Technologies That Can Detect Most Cancers Early with a Single Test

A New Path Forward— Systemic Early Detection

"There can be life after breast cancer. The prerequisite is early detection."
Ann Jillian

What is the most effective path forward for conquering cancer with our current knowledge and experience?

In this chapter, we will pause to scrupulously assess the progress and current status of cancer treatment, prevention, and early detection as detailed in previous chapters. I will then delve into our forthcoming endeavors in the quest to conquer cancer, underscoring the imperative of systemic early detection throughout the whole body to catch most cancer types early.

Metastatic Cancer Remains Largely Incurable

In the profound abyss of humanity's ongoing battle against cancer—a malignant force that has insidiously extended beyond its initial confines—we face a formidable adversary that remains complex and adaptive, consistently challenging our most sophisticated treatments.

Early cancer stages, typically Stages I and II, involve limited tumor size and spread. At these stages, cancer is confined to its origin, showing no signs of spreading to other body parts. During Stage I, the tumor is small and has not reached neighboring lymph nodes or distant areas, remaining within its organ of origin without invading deeper tissues. In Stage II, the cancer grows larger than in Stage I and may start affecting nearby tissues or lymph nodes. Localized cancers are often curable with surgery, and may require additional therapies like radiation or localized chemotherapy to eliminate all cancer cells.

Late-stage cancer, encompassing Stages III and IV, presents greater complexity and treatment challenges due to extensive spread. Stage III cancer may have infiltrated nearby tissues, organs, and lymph nodes but remains predominantly in the original area. Managing Stage III often requires a combination of treatments, including surgery, radiation, and systemic chemotherapy. Stage IV, or metastatic cancer, indicates that cancer cells have traveled through the lymphatic system or bloodstream to establish secondary tumors in distant organs such as the lungs, liver, bones, or brain. Stage IV cancer is generally incurable, focusing on palliative care to alleviate symptoms and enhance quality of life rather than pursuing curative treatments.

Metastatic cancer remains one of the most formidable challenges in medicine despite significant advancements in cancer treatment over recent decades. Although breakthroughs in targeted therapies, immunotherapies, and precision medicine have transformed cancer care and improved outcomes for many patients, metastatic cancer largely remains incurable.

Targeted therapies, which specifically attack molecular targets involved in cancer growth and progression, have shown efficacy in certain cancer types. For example, drugs targeting the EGFR mutation in lung cancer or HER2 in breast cancer have significantly improved survival rates for some patients. Immunotherapies, which leverage the body's immune system to combat cancer, have produced durable responses in some patients with advanced melanoma, lung cancer, and other malignancies. Precision medicine, which tailors treatment based on the genetic profile of a patient's tumor, has enabled more personalized and potentially effective treatment strategies.

However, metastatic cancer often finds a way to evade or resist these treatments due to tumor heterogeneity, adaptive mutations, and tumor microenvironment complexity. This enduring challenge of finding a cure compels us to adopt a new perspective in the fight against cancer, encompassing both prevention and early detection.

Decline in Cancer Mortality Rate in the US Primarily Due to Prevention and Early Detection

The collective efforts to translate knowledge about modifiable cancer risk factors and early detection by screening have borne significant fruits. The cancer mortality rate has declined significantly in the United States in recent decades. Between 1991 and 2019, the cancer death rate decreased by 32%, although the total number of cancer cases and deaths still rises.

The decline in the US cancer mortality rate is primarily due to reductions in smoking, advancements in early detection, and improvements in treatment. Let's review the significant contributions of cancer prevention and screening/early detection in the decline.

Contribution of Cancer Prevention

- **Tobacco Control.** Smoking, a major cause of cancer, especially lung cancer, has been aggressively targeted through comprehensive tobacco control measures. These measures include public smoking bans, higher taxes, advertising restrictions, and smoking cessation programs. As a result, adult smoking rates have dramatically decreased from 42% in 1965 to just 14% in 2019, according to the American Cancer Society. This decline has led to a 51%

reduction in lung cancer mortality among men and a 26% reduction among women between 1991 and 2018, as reported by the National Cancer Institute.

- **Vaccination.** The human papillomavirus (HPV), a significant cause of cervical, anal, and oropharyngeal cancers, has been effectively combated through the HPV vaccine. The Centers for Disease Control and Prevention (CDC) reports an 86% reduction in HPV infections among teenage girls from 2006 to 2017. This success, combined with diligent screening, has resulted in a 50% decrease in cervical cancer death rates from 1975 to 2018, marking a major public health victory.

- **Healthy Lifestyle.** Public health campaigns have emphasized the importance of healthy diets, regular physical activity, and healthy weight. These lifestyle changes are crucial for cancer prevention, as approximately 18% of cancer cases and 16% of cancer deaths in the United States are linked to excess body weight, poor nutrition, and physical inactivity.

- **Environmental and Occupational Safety.** Efforts to limit exposure to carcinogenic agents in the environment and workplace have made significant strides. Regulations reducing exposure to substances like asbestos have led to a marked decline in mesothelioma, a cancer closely associated with asbestos exposure.

Contribution of Early Detection

Early detection drastically improves survival outcomes. Cancers found in their early stages are typically more treatable and have higher survival rates. For example:

- **Breast Cancer Screening:** The 5-year survival rate for localized breast cancer is 99%, compared to 28% for cancer that has metastasized. The breast cancer death rate decreased by 40% from 1989 to 2017. This decline is attributed to the widespread adoption of mammography screening and improved treatments.

- **Colorectal Cancer Screening:** Early-stage colorectal cancer patients have a 5-year survival rate of 90%, which falls to about 14% for advanced-stage cancer. Colorectal cancer death rates dropped by 55% among men and 57% among women from 1970 to 2018. This decline is largely due to screening.

- **Lung Cancer Screening:** Patients with early-stage lung cancer have a 5-year survival rate of approximately 56%, versus only 5% for those diagnosed at a late stage. The reduction in lung cancer death rate is mainly due to decreased smoking rates, early detection, and treatment advancements.

- **Prostate Cancer Screening:** Prostate cancer death rates fell by about 52% from 1993 to 2018, thanks to PSA testing and advances in treatment.

In summary, the US's decline in cancer mortality rate underscores the power of prevention and early detection. These significant differences in localized and metastatic cancer survival rates underscore the crucial role of early detection.

The Barrier of Nonmodifiable Risk Factors in Cancer Prevention

In our ongoing battle against cancer, prevention has become a vital public health strategy to reduce its global incidence. Lifestyle changes such as quitting smoking, reducing alcohol consumption, improving diet, and increasing physical activity, alongside vaccinations against cancer-causing viruses like HPV and HBV and robust environmental policies, have all contributed to lowering cancer rates to some extent.

However, we face the major obstacle of nonmodifiable risk factors, including aging. As the global population ages, the incidence of cancer rises, highlighting the challenges in preventing the disease.

We are witnessing a significant demographic shift, with populations aging rapidly due to higher life expectancies and lower birth rates. According to the World Health Organization, the proportion of people over 60 will nearly double from 12% to 22% between 2015 and 2050.

Aging is the most significant risk factor for cancer, with most diagnoses occurring in individuals aged 65 and older. Consequently, the aging population is expected to increase the number of cancer cases, complicating efforts to reduce cancer incidence through prevention.

The link between aging and cancer is driven by several biological mechanisms that increase cancer risk as individuals age, including genetic mutations and weakened immune systems. Aging cells experience higher DNA damage and mutation rates due to exposure to carcinogens and inherent errors in cellular processes. Over time, the accumulation of these mutations can lead to cancer. As we age, the immune system becomes less effective at identifying and eliminating precancerous and cancerous cells.

While cancer prevention strategies that address modifiable risk factors can significantly reduce cancer incidence, aging presents an insurmountable challenge. This is evidenced by the continuous rise in cancer cases in the United States and globally. Thus, cancer prevention faces an insuperable barrier: **aging, the most significant yet non-modifiable risk factor**.

Significant Gaps in Early Detection

Early detection as a secondary cancer prevention becomes critical in the battle against cancer. However, early-stage, localized cancer is often asymptomatic, showing no noticeable symptoms until it advances. Localized cancers caught early are often curable through surgical removal or localized treatments like radiation.

Unfortunately, current early detection methods are limited to a few cancer types, such as breast, cervical, lung, and colorectal cancers, which can be effectively identified through established tests like mammograms, Pap smears, chest CT, and colonoscopies. These cancers benefit from well-publicized and widely implemented screening programs that have significantly lowered mortality rates through early detection and treatment.

Alarmingly, the majority of cancer deaths are caused by cancer types that lack recommended screening methods, including pancreatic, liver, ovarian, kidney, esophageal, and gastric cancers. This highlights critical gaps in our current early cancer detection efforts. **Thus, developing and adopting innovative early detection technologies have become imperative to fill the significant gap in cancer screening and early detection.**

A New Path Forward: Innovative Systemic Early Detection

The continuing global rise in cancer incidence and mortality underscores the overall ineffectiveness of current treatments, prevention, and early detection, as discussed earlier. Approximately 1.9 million new cancer cases emerged in 2022, and 609,360 lives were claimed by cancer in the United States during the same year.

Recent studies reveal an alarming increase in cancer rates among younger individuals, particularly those under 50 years old. Termed early-onset cancer, this trend spans various cancer types across multiple countries. In the United States, cancer diagnoses in adults under 50 have climbed from about 100 per 100,000 people in 2010 to 103 per 100,000 in 2019. Colorectal cancer rates have nearly doubled among young adults since the 1990s. Similarly, early-onset breast cancer is on the rise, with incidences increasing by almost 4% annually among U.S. women from 2016 to 2019. A global study analyzing data from 204 countries found a 79.1% increase in early-onset cancer cases from 1990 to 2019, with 3.26 million cases reported in 2019. Factors potentially driving this trend include rising obesity rates, higher consumption of processed foods, reduced physical activity, and increased exposure to environmental pollutants and carcinogens. The growing prevalence of early-onset cancers highlights the need for heightened cancer awareness and screening, even among younger populations.

The need for better cancer screening and early detection is widely recognized. As Bruce Ratner and Adam Bonislawski aptly stated in their recent book, "Catching cancer early remains the single best way to combat a disease that is the second-leading killer in both the US and worldwide. But the vast majority of resources in the fight against cancer are devoted to relatively ineffective late-stage treatments."

"Early detection and prevention are currently the biggest unmet needs in cancer," said Marcel van den Brink, M.D., Ph.D., president of City of Hope Los Angeles and City of Hope National Medical Center. "Finding cancers early or preventing them in the first place can literally mean the difference between life and death."

Given the substantial gaps in current single-site cancer screening tests, innovative early detection technologies capable of screening most cancer types with a single test are urgently needed.

Over the past decade, I have redirected the focus of my research team from finding a cure to developing new cancer detection methods and preventive cancer vaccines. In the forthcoming chapters, I will explore the latest breakthroughs in cancer detection technologies and advocate for the timely adoption of innovative systemic screening tests for the early detection of most cancer types with a single test.

Sensing the Tell-tale Signal of a Hidden Tumor

CHAPTER SIX

"Cancer isn't what kills us. It is cancer caught at later stages that kills people,"
Cristian Tomasetti

Is it feasible to detect most cancer types early with just one single test?

I pondered this possibility a decade ago.

With each passing year, the risk of insidious cancer, poised to strike without warning, increases. Tales of seemingly healthy friends ravaged by the disease's stealthy strike have unsettled me.

Early detection was crucial, yet our screening methods felt woefully inadequate. While dedicated single-site screening tests could identify threats like breast, cervical, colorectal, lung, and prostate cancers, the majority of malignancies remained hidden until they reached incurable late stages—where over 75% of cancer deaths occurred.

It was disheartening to realize we lacked systemic screening tools to preemptively identify cancer's cellular subversions before they evolved into full-blown diseases. Our existing tools were akin to searching for needles in haystacks, blind to the incremental gene mutations silently giving rise to malignancy.

Over a decade ago, this existential dread spurred me to pivot my research toward developing better early detection technologies.

My quest led me to a 2001 paper by Dr. Gabriella Sozzi's Italian team, which explored circulating tumor DNA in lung cancer patients' blood plasmas as a potential diagnostic biomarker (*Cancer Res.* 2001). Their study of 84 patients and 43 healthy controls revealed that elevated cell-free circulating DNA levels could distinguish cancer cases, even in early stages, and tracked disease progression. This promising study suggested that molecular liquid biopsy tests analyzing blood for tumor DNA could detect malignancies far earlier than conventional methods.

This promise was bolstered in 2005 when the esteemed Dr. Bert Vogelstein of Johns Hopkins University reported detecting mutant DNA from colorectal cancers in patient blood samples (*Proc Natl Acad Sci USA.* 2005). The concept ignited intense interest across oncology.

Inspired, I made efforts to develop our own circulating tumor DNA sequencing tests in collaboration with physicians. After years of laborious effort, we demonstrated the ability to identify lung cancer driver mutations in early-stage patients simply from a blood draw by sequencing blood circulating tumor DNA (ctDNA) in 2014 (*Sci Rep* 2014, 2016). We had found the needle in the haystack.

Let us now review the history and recent advancements in ctDNA tests that are capable of detecting early signals of hidden tumors. These groundbreaking liquid biopsy tests can effectively identify most cancer types in asymptomatic, healthy individuals through a single blood test.

Development of Circulating Tumor DNA (ctDNA) Tests

The evolution of cell-free DNA (cfDNA) and circulating tumor DNA (ctDNA) detection technology represents an extraordinary journey, intertwining advancements in molecular biology, cancer research, and diagnostic methodologies. This breakthrough exemplifies the relentless pursuit of innovation in biological and medical science.

ctDNA testing, often called liquid biopsy, marks a groundbreaking leap in cancer diagnostics and monitoring. The progression of ctDNA technology, from its conceptual origins to contemporary clinical applications, embraces numerous technical advancements.

Early Discoveries and Conceptual Foundations: The concept of ctDNA dates back to the mid-20th century. In 1948, the French scientists Mandel and Metais first reported the presence of free nucleic acids in the bloodstream. However, the significance of circulating DNA in cancer wasn't recognized until the 1970s and 1980s. During these decades, researchers observed elevated levels of circulating DNA in cancer patients, suggesting its potential as a biomarker for malignancies. In 1989, Swiss researchers Stroun and Anker at the University of Geneva made a landmark discovery by identifying tumor-derived DNA in the blood of cancer patients, laying the foundation for ctDNA as a cancer biomarker.

Technological Advances Enabling ctDNA Detection: A critical technological breakthrough came with the development of polymerase chain reaction (PCR) by American scientist Kary Mullis in 1983, who was awarded the Nobel Prize in Chemistry in 1993. PCR technology allowed for amplifying and detecting small DNA quantities with heightened sensitivity and specificity, paving the way for clinical liquid biopsies. In the early 2000s, Bert Vogelstein and colleagues introduced digital PCR, a highly sensitive method for quantifying ctDNA. Next-generation sequencing (NGS) further revolutionized the field by enabling comprehensive analysis of genetic mutations and alterations in ctDNA, identifying cancer-related genetic changes. DNA sequencing began with the groundbreaking discovery of the DNA structure by James Watson and Francis Crick in 1953.

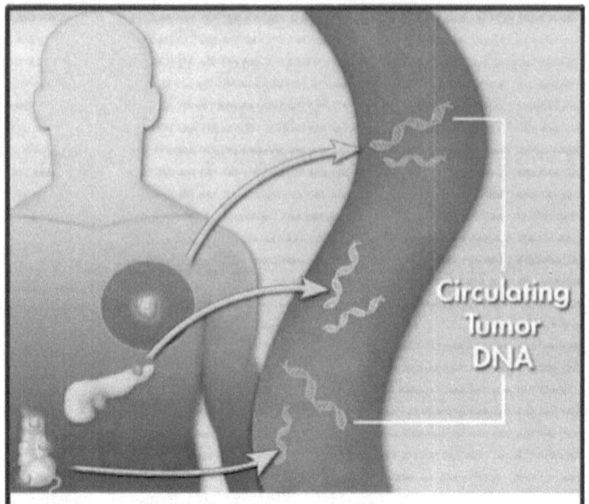

Tumors shed pieces of DNA into the
bloodstream as circulating tumor DNA
(ctDNA) that can be detected.
Source: NCI

This fundamental understanding set the stage to decode the DNA sequence. In 1977, British scientist Fred Sanger developed the chain termination DNA sequencing method, known as Sanger sequencing, which became the gold standard due to its accuracy and reliability. Sanger won his second Nobel Prize in 1980 for his contribution to DNA sequencing. The advent of NGS in the mid-2000s dramatically increased sequencing throughput while reducing costs. Technologies like Illumina's sequencing by synthesis (SBS) and Roche's 454 pyrosequencing enabled the simultaneous sequencing of millions of DNA fragments. Shankar Balasubramanian and David Klenerman, founders of Solexa (later acquired by Illumina), developed the SBS technology that became the cornerstone of NGS platforms.

The ability to detect and analyze ctDNA in the bloodstream marks a revolutionary advancement in cancer diagnostics. ctDNA tests provide a non-invasive glimpse into the genetic essence of malignancies. Cell-free DNA (cfDNA) refers to DNA fragments naturally released into the bloodstream from dying cells. However, circulating tumor DNA (ctDNA) holds particular significance as these fragments originate from tumor cells, carrying the distinct mutation signatures of cancer.

Tumors continuously shed DNA fragments with their unique mutation and methylation patterns into the bloodstream. By detecting and interpreting ctDNA, clinicians can non-invasively identify the genetic disruptions driving a patient's cancer.

Research has shown that ctDNA levels in the blood correlate with tumor burden, fluctuating as cancers progress or respond to treatments. Specific mutation patterns and fragment characteristics distinguish a cancer patient's ctDNA from the cfDNA released by healthy cells.

Imagine the power of a simple blood test to detect cancer's presence and reveal its specific type and optimal treatments. This is the compelling promise of ctDNA. Instead of invasive biopsies or waiting for symptoms, these tests scan the bloodstream for DNA fragments shed by emerging tumor cells.

With the capability to identify cancer's earliest molecular signs, ctDNA testing dramatically increases the chances of a cure by catching the disease before it spreads. ctDNA testing brings a new ray of hope where it's most urgently needed, extending far beyond mere detection. By deciphering cancer's genetic essence, ctDNA analysis facilitates precision therapies tailored to each patient's tumor profile, eliminating the need for traumatic trial-and-error treatments. This approach ensures personalized therapies that maximize efficacy and minimize toxicity. Moreover, ctDNA's sharp detection skills allow for vigilant monitoring, quickly alerting to any cancer recurrence and offering reassurance by reducing the agonizing uncertainty of potential relapse.

The journey of ctDNA technology from its initial stages to its current sophisticated applications showcases the tremendous strides made in cancer diagnostics and the indomitable spirit of scientific inquiry and innovation.

Now, let's review the clinical applications of ctDNA tests for cancer detection.

ctDNA Tests for Detecting Mutations as Companion Diagnostics

In 2014, the FDA approved the first liquid biopsy test, Roche's EGFR Mutation ctDNA Test, for detecting EGFR mutations in lung cancer patients. This approval marked a milestone in accepting ctDNA testing in clinical practice as companion diagnostics.

Here is a summary of FDA-approved ctDNA tests to guide cancer treatment:

- Cobas EGFR Mutation Test: This PCR-based test detects EGFR gene mutations in ctDNA from lung cancer patients. It is approved as a companion diagnostic to select lung cancer patients for treatment with specific EGFR tyrosine kinase inhibitors.

- Therascreen PIK3CA Kit: This PCR test identifies 11 PIK3CA genetic mutations in ctDNA from breast cancer patients. It is approved to select breast cancer patients for treatment with the PI3K inhibitor drug alpelisib.

- Guardant360 CDx: This NGS-based liquid biopsy test analyzes 55 genes in ctDNA. It is approved as a companion diagnostic for several targeted therapies and for tumor mutation profiling in certain cancer types.

- F1 Liquid CDx: Another NGS-based ctDNA test approved as a companion diagnostic for tumor profiling across various solid tumors.

The advancements in ctDNA testing stand as a testament to the progress in precision cancer treatment, promising a future where personalized therapies are the norm for pinpointing targetable cancer mutations.

Challenges of ctDNA Tests for Early Cancer Screening

ctDNA holds immense promise for non-invasive, universal early cancer detection, with the potential to profoundly reshape early diagnosis and intervention. This technology identifies tumor DNA signatures shed by tumor cells into the bloodstream, signifying a paradigm shift from single-site cancer detection to systemic detection for most cancer types with a single blood test.

However, early cancer detection through ctDNA testing faces significant challenges, particularly in early stage I/II cancers where ctDNA levels are extremely low. Detecting these sparse ctDNA molecules amid the background noise of cell-free DNA from normal cells requires ultra-sensitive technologies like massively deep next-generation sequencing, capable of parsing individual mutations with high resolution. Achieving the required depth, often exceeding 10,000x coverage, imposes substantial costs and computational demands. It necessitates sophisticated techniques to enhance signal accuracy while minimizing artifacts and errors inherent in such deep DNA sequencing.

Moreover, cancer's genetic diversity presents another challenge. Tumors from different tissues possess distinct mutation signatures, reflecting their unique lineage. Even within a single patient, cancers exhibit extensive heterogeneity as they evolve, diversifying with each new mutation.

Thus, detecting genetic mutations in ctDNA for identifying early-stage cancer has been hindered by the minuscule levels of tumor DNA in early malignancies and the vast diversity of mutations across different cancers. New technologies are needed to unlock the full potential of ctDNA testing for early cancer detection.

Breakthrough: Detecting Methylation Patterns in ctDNA for Early Cancer Detection

Basic cancer research reveals that DNA methylation is a crucial biochemical process in which a methyl group (CH_3) is added to DNA, primarily at cytosine bases followed by guanine bases, known as CpG sites. This process is essential for regulating gene expression and maintaining genomic stability. By attaching methyl groups to the promoter regions of genes, cells can effectively suppress gene transcription, turning genes "off" when not required, thereby ensuring proper cellular function and development.

In cancer cells, methylation patterns often become disrupted, resulting in either hypermethylation or hypomethylation. Hypermethylation in the promoter regions of tumor suppressor genes can silence these critical genes, leading to uncontrolled cell growth. This alteration can impact cell cycle regulation, DNA repair, and apoptosis pathways, thereby contributing to tumorigenesis. On the other hand, global hypomethylation can activate oncogenes, promoting cancer progression through unchecked cellular proliferation and survival. Thus, these altered methylation patterns in cancer cells can serve as valuable biomarkers for early cancer detection.

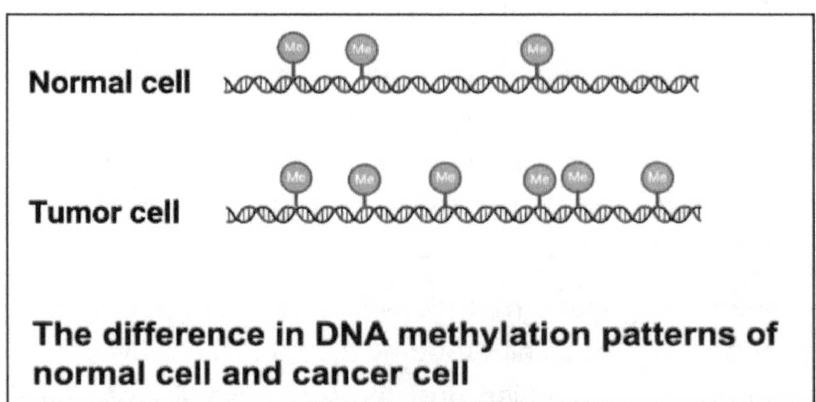

The difference in DNA methylation patterns of normal cell and cancer cell

Recent DNA sequencing and computational analysis advances have made methylation profiling a powerful diagnostic tool. Next-generation technologies can map millions of methylation sites across ctDNA molecules while sophisticated algorithms identify the distinct patterns in ctDNA.

One such ctDNA test, developed by the biotech company GRAIL, uses this DNA methylation detection approach. It examines methylation patterns on ctDNA to detect cancers before symptoms arise. From enriching for methylation hotspots to high-resolution sequencing and algorithmically interpreting complex data, this liquid biopsy workflow reveals methylation aberrations indicative of early tumorigenesis. It differentiates cancerous from non-cancerous tissues based on their unique methylation signatures.

While evolving, ctDNA methylation profiling represents a transformative frontier—a glimpse into cancer's earliest stages through a simple blood draw. As technologies advance, this liquid biopsy method could revolutionize screening paradigms and pave the way for the systemic early detection of most cancer types with a single blood test.

Tracing the Origins of ctDNA

DNA methylation patterns are unique modifications that influence gene expression. These patterns are tissue-specific, meaning different tissues and organs in the body exhibit distinct DNA methylation signatures. The methylation patterns in ctDNA mirror the methylation status of the tissues from which they originate. For instance, ctDNA derived from liver cells will possess a different methylation signature than lung cells. By analyzing these methylation patterns, scientists can determine the tissue or organ of origin for the ctDNA found in a blood sample. This uniqueness serves as the foundation for tracing the origin of ctDNA.

The ability to trace the tissue origin of ctDNA is particularly valuable for early cancer detection in asymptomatic individuals. Tumors release ctDNA into the bloodstream, and the methylation patterns of this ctDNA can reveal information about the type and location of the cancer. For example, if ctDNA in the blood exhibits methylation patterns characteristic of the pancreas, it suggests that the ctDNA originates from a pancreatic tumor.

Furthermore, the tissue-specific methylation patterns of ctDNA can differentiate between various tumor types arising within the same organ or distinguish primary tumors from metastases. This detailed information enhances the accuracy of cancer detection and facilitates more personalized and effective intervention.

In summary, the distinct DNA methylation patterns found in different tissues and organs allow for tracing the origin of blood ctDNA. This capability is a powerful asset in liquid biopsy, offering insights into the tissue-specific origins of ctDNA, which are crucial for early cancer detection, diagnosis, and monitoring.

Recent Advances in ctDNA Detection Technologies

There are many advances in improving the sensitivity and specificity of ctDNA tests. A frontier known as fragmentomics can potentially enhance liquid biopsy testing by detecting cancer's most elusive beginnings. Cancerous cells release DNA fragments with distinct length patterns compared to healthy cells due to differences in enzymes and chromatin packaging. Fragmentomics leverages this by analyzing all cell-free DNA molecules' physical characteristics and fragmentation signatures through whole-genome sequencing. By examining these genome-wide fragmentation codes, machine learning algorithms can identify the subtle fingerprints of malignancy, even in the earliest stages of the disease. This methodology shows promise in significantly enhancing the sensitivity of tests to detect early-stage tumors that may go undetected by conventional ctDNA assays. Additionally, fragmentomics eliminates the need for pre-specified gene panels, offering a cost-effective solution for comprehensive multi-cancer screening.

Other advancements and strategies are being explored to increase the sensitivity of ctDNA detection by minimizing its degradation. Researchers have demonstrated that they can temporarily boost the amount of ctDNA in the blood of cancer patients, thereby improving the sensitivity of liquid biopsy tests. This approach involves administering agents that increase the release of ctDNA from tumor cells into the bloodstream, raising the ctDNA concentration and making it easier to detect.

Continuous advancements in ctDNA detection technologies are expected to enhance liquid biopsies' sensitivity, accuracy, and clinical applicability. These innovations could usher in a new era of cancer early detection and interception, illuminating the faintest traces of malignancy for optimal early detection and intervention.

Blood ctDNA Test for Colorectal Cancer Detection

Guardant Health's Shield blood ctDNA test has been recommended for FDA approval for screening colorectal cancer in adults aged 45 and older at average risk in 2024. Shield ctDNA test marks a significant advance in the application of ctDNA tests for cancer screening. Shield test focuses on analyzing genomic and epigenomic changes in blood ctDNA. The extensive ECLIPSE study underscored the test's efficacy, encompassing over 20,000 participants. The results revealed that Shield achieved an 83% sensitivity and a 90% specificity for detecting colorectal cancer. Although its sensitivity for precancerous lesions was lower at 13%, Shield remains a valuable addition to existing screening strategies. While Shield is not meant to replace colonoscopy, it serves as a complement to current screening options. Its non-invasive nature and simplicity—a mere blood draw—make it an appealing alternative for those hesitant about invasive procedures. As a blood-based test, Shield offers a more convenient screening option, which could help overcome obstacles linked with traditional colonoscopy and stool-based tests.

Systemic Early Cancer Detection with a Single ctDNA Test-- Clinical Validation

Galleri MCED test, developed by a biotech company, GRAIL, represents a significant milestone in pursuing early detection of multiple cancers through a single blood ctDNA test. This breakthrough offers new hope for identifying cancers at an early stage, potentially preventing their insidious progression via early intervention.

Multi-cancer Early Detection (MCED) tests like Galleri can detect signals from over 50 types of cancer through a single blood sample. This test is designed to identify a variety of cancers, many of which currently lack screening methods. Here is a list of representative cancer types that a single Galleri MCED blood test can detect:

Cancers Detectable by Galleri's MCED Blood Test

Cancer Type	Cancer Type	Cancer Type	Cancer Type
Bladder Cancer	Breast Cancer	Cervical Cancer	Colorectal Cancer
Esophageal Cancer	Gastric Cancer	Head and Neck Cancer	Kidney Cancer
Liver Cancer	Lung Cancer	Lymphoma	Melanoma
Multiple Myeloma	Ovarian Cancer	Pancreatic Cancer	Prostate Cancer
Sarcoma	Thyroid Cancer	Gallbladder Cancer	Bile Duct Cancer
Endometrial Cancer	Uterine Cancer	Small Intestine Cancer	Unknown Primary Cancer

Validating ctDNA testing clinically is crucial to ensure these ctDNA tests reliably detect cancer in both symptomatic and asymptomatic individuals. This rigorous process involves a range of clinical trials, including validation trials to assess effectiveness, early detection trials to evaluate the ability to catch cancer early, population-based trials to test performance across diverse cohorts, and longitudinal studies to measure long-term impacts. Some key clinical trials, such as the CCGA, PATHFINDE, and SYMPLIFY studies, are described here.

The CCGA Study: A Multi-Center Trial of Galleri's MCED Test

The CCGA (Circulating Cell-free Genome Atlas) study is a comprehensive and longitudinal initiative to validate the utility of blood Galleri's MCED ctDNA test to detect multiple cancer types. This study involves 15,000 participants across 142 sites in the US and Canada, encompassing a diverse group, including newly diagnosed cancer patients and a group without known cancer diagnoses. Participants are monitored annually for up to five years, providing valuable longitudinal data. The primary goal is to evaluate MCED ctDNA testing's ability to detect and pinpoint cancer origins using advanced genomic sequencing and machine learning to analyze ctDNA's methylation patterns.

The clinical validation of MCED ctDNA testing focuses on its sensitivity and specificity for cancer detection. Sensitivity measures the test's ability to identify patients with cancer, while specificity assesses its accuracy in excluding those who do not have cancer.

Results from a substudy included 4,077 participants in an independent validation set (cancer: n = 2,823; non-cancer: n = 1,254, with non-cancer status confirmed at one-year follow-up). Here are the key findings of this substudy (*Ann Oncol.* 2021):

- The specificity for cancer signal detection was 99.5%.

- Overall sensitivity for cancer signal detection was 51.5%, varying by stage. Sensitivity for stages I-III in 12 cancer types, which account for about two-thirds of annual US cancer deaths, was 67.6%. For all cancer types, it was 40.7%.

Sensitivity varies significantly among different cancers, being higher for lethal cancers such as liver and pancreatic and lower for others like prostate and breast, which may not shed as much DNA into the bloodstream.

The PATHFINDER Study: A Prospective, Multi-Center Research Endeavor in Asymptomatic Populations for Early Detection

The PATHFINDER study is a prospective, multi-center study designed to evaluate the utility of GRAIL's MCED ctDNA test for systemic early cancer detection in a real-world setting. The study enrolled 6,662 asymptomatic adults aged 50 and older to undergo the MCED tests.

Key results of this clinical study were published in *The Lancet* in 2023 and are summarized here:

- Detection Rates: A cancer signal was detected in 1.4% of participants, with cancer subsequently confirmed in 0.5% of the total cohort.

- Cancer Stage at Detection: Nearly half (48%) of the cancers detected were at early stages (stage I or II), enhancing the potential for curative treatment.

- Prediction Accuracy of Cancer Signal Origin: The MCED test demonstrated 97% accuracy in predicting the cancer signal origin (CSO), enabling precise and targeted diagnostic follow-ups.

- Types of Cancers Detected: Significantly, 74% of the detected cancers were types that lack recommended screening options, such as cancers of the bile duct, small intestine, and pancreas, often undiagnosed until later stages.

The PATHFINDER study highlights the transformative potential of the MCED test in cancer screening, which is capable of early detection across multiple cancer types, including those without current screening protocols in asymptomatic individuals.

The SYMPLIFY Study: Large-Scale Trial in Symptomatic Populations for Cancer Detection

The SYMPLIFY study is another key trial to evaluate MCED tests' application in symptomatic populations. This prospective, multi-center trial aims to evaluate the effectiveness of MCED tests in detecting cancer in individuals presenting with suspicious symptoms. The study assesses the test's diagnostic accuracy and clinical utility in a symptomatic cohort (*Lancet Oncol.* 2023).

While the PATHFINDER study explored GRAIL's MCED blood test for screening and early detection, the SYMPLIFY study, sponsored by the University of Oxford, investigated its use in confirming cancer in patients with suspected symptoms. It enrolled 6,238 patients across England and Wales who were urgently referred by their doctors for advanced imaging tests like CT scans or endoscopies due to concerning symptoms.

The MCED test demonstrated exceptional specificity of 98.4%, meaning very few healthy patients received false positives. Additionally, when it signaled the presence of cancer, it accurately predicted the tumor's origin or location 85.2% of the time based on DNA signatures, enabling doctors to pursue appropriate diagnostic workups rapidly.

The SYMPLIFY study identified cancer in 323 patients, with 244 confirmed as true positives through standard diagnostic methods. The MCED test demonstrated an overall sensitivity of 66.3% for detecting cancer across all stages, increasing from 24.2% in early-stage I to an impressive 95.3% in late-stage IV cancers.

Sir Harpal Kumar, President of GRAIL Europe, highlighted, "The SYMPLIFY data confirm the potential benefit of methylation-based MCED blood tests as a diagnostic aid for symptomatic patients. These promising results will guide our development of an optimized classifier for use in patients suspected of having cancer."

In summary, GRAIL's MCED ctDNA test, evaluated in the CCGA, PATHFINDER, and SYMPLIFY clinical studies, demonstrates its specificity and sensitivity in detecting most cancer types with a single blood test.

High Positive Predictive Value of ctDNA Tests

In cancer screening, one critical measure stands out as a beacon of a test's reliability and utility: the Positive Predictive Value (PPV). This metric is not just another statistic; it serves as the compass guiding us through the intricate landscape of early cancer detection. PPV reveals how often a positive test result indeed indicates the presence of cancer, helping to avert unnecessary anxiety and follow-up procedures for patients.

Imagine being a navigator charting a course through treacherous waters. Working with PPV in cancer screening is akin to this. PPV is your North Star, indicating the likelihood that a positive screening result genuinely signifies disease. The formula, akin to your sextant, is:

$$PPV = TP / (TP + FP)$$

TP represents True Positives—people correctly identified as having cancer—and FP stands for False Positives—those incorrectly flagged.

A high PPV indicates that your test is a skilled navigator, accurately distinguishing those with cancer from those without. Conversely, a low PPV is like following a faulty compass, potentially leading to false positives and unnecessary follow-up examinations. A high PPV fosters more confident clinical decision-making, allowing healthcare providers to recommend further diagnostic procedures or treatments more confidently.

Impressively High PPV of the MCED ctDNA Tests

Galleri MCED Test

The PPV of the Galleri MCED ctDNA Test, capable of identifying over 50 types of cancer, stands at an impressive 38% in asymptomatic individuals (PATHFINDER Study) and 75.5% in the symptomatic patient population (SYMPLIFY Study).

The Galleri MCED Test has a PPV of 38% in asymptomatic individuals, indicating that about 38 out of 100 individuals with a "Cancer Signal Detected" result are expected to receive a confirmed cancer diagnosis with follow-up tests such as a biopsy. This high PPV is particularly significant given the test's broad applicability across multiple cancer types, which currently lack effective early detection methods.

Moreover, the test boasts a 99.5% specificity with a low false-positive rate of 0.5%, which is highly accurate in determining when no cancer-related signals are present in a sample. The low false-positive rate of 0.5% means that in approximately 200 people without cancer, only one person would receive a false-positive result.

Other MCED Tests

Many companies are developing various MCED tests. Here's a summary of the PPV of other MCED tests:

SPOT-MAS: This test has a high PPV of 60% in clinical trials. Utilizing NGS and artificial intelligence, SPOT-MAS analyzes methylation profiles and multiple ctDNA features to detect up to 10 common cancers at their earliest stages.

CancerSEEK: With a PPV of 19.4% in clinical trials, CancerSEEK integrates liquid biopsy techniques with detecting specific protein biomarkers linked to various cancers. It targets ctDNA mutations and cancer-related proteins to identify eight types of cancer, including ovarian, liver, and pancreatic cancers.

SeekInCare: Demonstrating a PPV of 11.5% in clinical trials, SeekInCare detects multiple cancer types by identifying abnormal DNA fragments in the blood.

Comparing with PPV of Current Cancer Screening Tests

Let's review and compare the PPV of the MCED ctDNA Test with current cancer screening tests.

- **Mammography for Breast Cancer:** The PPV of the well-established mammography is ~10% for women in their 40s and ~30% for women over 50, significantly lower than 38% of Galleri's MCED ctDNA tests.

- **Low-Dose Computed Tomography (LDCT) for Lung Cancer:** The PPV of LDCT for lung cancer screening is about 4% to 5% in high-risk populations, such as heavy smokers, with much lower PPV compared to the Galleri test.

- **Fecal Occult Blood Test (FOBT) and Fecal Immunochemical Test (FIT) for Colorectal Cancer:** The PPV of FOBT and FIT for colorectal cancer ranges from 5% to 10%, much lower PPV compared to the Galleri test.

- **Colonoscopy:** Considered the gold standard for detecting colorectal cancer and precancerous polyps, colonoscopy is an invasive procedure that can remove polyps as an intervention. Surprisingly, the exact PPV of colonoscopy for cancer screening is not available.

- **Prostate-Specific Antigen (PSA) Test for Prostate Cancer:** The PPV of the PSA test is approximately 25% to 30% for men over 50, which was lower than the Galleri test.

In summary, the Galleri MCED ctDNA test demonstrates a significant advantage in early cancer detection compared to other standard screening tests, with a high PPV of 38% in asymptomatic individuals and 75.5% in this symptomatic patient population. Since PPV is a crucial metric in assessing the effectiveness of cancer screening tests, the high PPV demonstrates that positive results of MCED ctDNA tests are reliable indicators of cancer in asymptomatic individuals.

Pitfalls of ctDNA Tests for Systemic Early Detection

While the promise of early cancer detection through MCED ctDNA technology is enticing, engaging in open discussions regarding its potential drawbacks and challenges is vital.

False Positives and Negatives. Although the Galleri MCED test has reportedly achieved a false-positive rate of less than 1%, false positives, which incorrectly suggest the presence of cancer, remain a concern. Cancer screening aims to achieve an optimal balance between high specificity and high sensitivity (its ability to identify those with cancer correctly). The ramifications of false positives extend beyond the immediate psychological effects on patients; they also raise broader concerns regarding healthcare resource utilization and the cost-effectiveness of cancer screening programs. Lowering the rate of false positives further can alleviate the clinical burden and costs tied to unnecessary follow-up diagnostic procedures, ultimately enhancing the efficiency and effectiveness of systemic cancer screening with ctDNA tests.

Concerns of Over-Diagnosis and Over-Treatment. Over-diagnosis occurs when a screening test identifies a cancer that is unlikely to cause symptoms or death during a person's lifetime. This can result in over-treatment, where patients undergo unnecessary medical interventions that may lead to significant side effects, impacting their quality of life. The challenge lies in distinguishing between aggressive tumors that require prompt intervention and indolent cancers that may never manifest clinically. Concerns regarding over-diagnosis and over-treatment are substantial for systemic cancer screening. However, GRAIL's MCED test was shown to detect more aggressive cancers preferentially. The test exhibits decreased sensitivity for indolent cancers, such as thyroid and encapsulated prostate cancer, thereby reducing the risk of over-diagnosis and unnecessary treatment. Nevertheless, further studies are needed to enhance the likelihood of identifying high-mortality cancers that necessitate timely intervention, ultimately improving patient outcomes without escalating medical care unnecessarily.

Ethical Considerations and Implementation. The ethical implications surrounding ctDNA tests revolve around their potential psychological impact on patients, the economic ramifications of widespread screening, and the clinical value of early cancer detection. A crucial question is whether identifying early-stage cancers in the blood genuinely benefits patients—especially when weighing the health economics of making such tests affordably accessible to a broad population versus targeting a narrower high-risk group.

Addressing these complexities requires a nuanced understanding of cancer biology and the development of screening technologies that are both sensitive and specific enough to identify which cancers pose an immediate threat. Moreover, it necessitates ongoing dialogue among healthcare providers, patients, and policymakers to ensure that ctDNA screening technologies are implemented to maximize benefits while minimizing harm.

Continued research and development are essential for refining these tests and enhancing their specificity, sensitivity, and clinical utility. Individuals considering an MCED ctDNA test, such as the Galleri test, should carefully weigh the benefits against the risks, taking into account personal health history, cancer risk factors, and the potential implications of the test results.

Landscape of MCED Test Companies

In the rapidly evolving field of cancer diagnostics, the development and clinical application of MCED ctDNA tests have become a focal point for researchers and clinicians. With the advent of MCED tests like the Galleri test by GRAIL, the landscape of cancer screening and detection is poised for significant transformation.

As briefly described below, several companies are leading the charge in developing ctDNA tests for cancer detection. These entities are leveraging the potential of ctDNA and other biomarkers to identify cancer at its earliest stages, employing a variety of innovative approaches and technologies:

- **Grail (Menlo Park, California):** Founded in January 2016 as a spin-off from Illumina, Grail was established by notable figures, including Jeffrey Huber (former Google senior executive), Jay Flatley (former CEO of Illumina), Rick Klausner (former Director of the National Cancer Institute), and Rafael Bejar (expert in hematologic malignancies and cancer genomics). Grail is renowned for its Galleri MCED test, which can identify over 50 types of cancers from a single blood draw. The test utilizes advanced NGS and machine learning to detect ctDNA associated with various cancers. Galleri has undergone extensive clinical validation, including the PATHFINDER studies, proving its effectiveness in early cancer detection. Grail's mission is to transform cancer care by making early detection accessible and effective, ultimately reducing cancer mortality through timely interventions.

- **Guardant Health (Redwood City, California):** Founded in 2012 by AmirAli Talasaz and Helmy Eltoukhy, Guardant Health specializes in developing liquid biopsy tests that analyze ctDNA for cancer detection and treatment monitoring. Their flagship product, Guardant360, is widely used for comprehensive genomic profiling of cancer patients to guide therapy decisions. The company is expanding its portfolio to include early-detection tests like Guardant Reveal, which focuses on minimal residual disease (MRD) and early detection of colorectal cancer. In

2024, Guardant Health's Shield blood ctDNA test was recommended for FDA approval to screen colorectal cancer in adults.

- **Foundation Medicine (Cambridge, Massachusetts)**. A leading biotechnology company was founded in 2010 by experts including Dr. Eric Lander, Dr. Levi Garraway, and Dr. Michael Pellini. The company specializes in molecular diagnostics for cancer, utilizing NGS technology to offer comprehensive genomic profiling tests. Their flagship product, FoundationOne® CDx, analyzes 324 genes associated with cancer to identify genetic mutations and genomic signatures like microsatellite instability and tumor mutational burden, which are crucial for guiding personalized cancer treatment. They also offer FoundationOne® Liquid CDx, a blood-based test that detects ctDNA, and FoundationOne® Heme, tailored for hematologic cancers. The company became a subsidiary of Roche in 2018.

- **Exact Sciences (Madison, Wisconsin):** Founded in 1995 by Stanley Lapidus, a pioneer in DNA-based diagnostics, Exact Sciences is best known for Cologuard, a non-invasive stool-based DNA test for colorectal cancer screening. The company also collaborates with Johns Hopkins University on the CancerSEEK test, a liquid biopsy designed to detect multiple cancer types by analyzing ctDNA and protein biomarkers. CancerSEEK is part of Exact Sciences' broader initiative to integrate early cancer detection into routine clinical care.

- **Seekln Inc. (San Diego, California):** Founded by Dr. Mao Mao, an expert in cancer genomics and early detection, Seekln Inc. developed the SeekInCare® liquid biopsy test, which aims to detect various cancers at early stages by identifying ctDNA in blood samples. The company focuses on making early cancer detection accessible and reliable through advancements in genomics and bioinformatics.

- **Gene Solutions (Ho Chi Minh City, Vietnam):** Co-founded by Dr. Phan Toan Thang, an expert in regenerative medicine and genetic testing, Gene Solutions offers the SPOT-MAS™ test, an MCED test that utilizes NGS and artificial intelligence (AI) to examine the methylation profiles of ctDNA for detecting multiple types of cancer at an early stage.

- **Burning Rock Biotech (Guangzhou, China):** Founded by Yusheng Han, an expert in genomic sequencing and cancer diagnostics, it developed the OverC™ test, which uses NGS to analyze ctDNA in blood samples, enabling the early detection of multiple cancer types.

- **StageZero Life Sciences (Richmond, Ontario):** Founded by a team of experts in genomics and early cancer detection, including Dr. Howard I. Manis, StageZero Life Sciences developed Aristotle®, a test designed to screen for multiple cancer types by analyzing ctDNA and other biomarkers in the blood.

- **Geneseeq (Toronto, Ontario):** Geneseeq developed the CanScan™ test. This test uses low-depth whole-genome sequencing on ctDNA to detect early cancer signals with high specificity and the ability to predict the tissue of origin of cancers, helping guide personalized treatment strategies.

- **Delfi (Baltimore, Maryland):** Founded by Dr. Victor Velculescu, a pioneer in cancer genomics, Delfi analyzes DNA fragmentation patterns in blood samples, which can indicate the presence of cancer. This approach offers a novel method for early cancer detection, providing valuable insights into the molecular characteristics of tumors.

- **Freenome (South San Francisco, California):** Founded by Gabriel Otte, Riley Ennis, and Michael Otte, Freenome combines ctDNA analysis with other biomarkers in its blood tests to detect early cancer. The company's proprietary platform integrates machine learning with multiomics to improve the accuracy and effectiveness of early detection tests.

- **Genetron Health (Beijing, China):** Founded by Sizhen Wang, an expert in precision oncology and genomics, Genetron Health developed a comprehensive screening platform that detects a broad spectrum of ctDNA alterations, offering detailed genetic profiles of cancers to guide personalized treatment approaches and improve early detection.

- **Ajinomoto (Tokyo, Japan):** Ajinomoto Co., Inc., a global leader in food and biotechnology, developed the AminoIndex Cancer Screening (AICS®) test, which analyzes amino acid concentrations in blood samples. Changes in these concentrations can indicate the presence of certain types of cancer, making AICS® a valuable tool in routine health checks and early cancer detection in Japan.

- **Datar Cancer Genetics (Bayreuth, Germany):** Founded by Rajan Datar, an entrepreneur, Datar Cancer Genetics developed the TruCheck™ test, a non-invasive blood-based screening test that detects circulating tumor cells (CTCs) to identify early-stage cancers. TruCheck™ is designed to provide a reliable and early diagnosis, even for cancers that are typically hard to detect.

- **Carcimun Biotech (Garmisch-Partenkirchen, Germany):** Founded by a team of oncologists and researchers specializing in cancer immunotherapy, Carcimun Biotech developed the Carcimun-test, which focuses on detecting cancer through immune response analysis. The test evaluates specific immune markers in the blood that

> indicate cancerous activity, offering another non-invasive method for early cancer detection.

- **EG BioMed (Taipei, Taiwan):** Founded by Dr. Ethan Shen, EG BioMed developed cfDNA methylation analysis for early cancer detection. It established Taiwan's first cfDNA genome-wide methylation database and integrated it with the US Cancer Genome Atlas, using big data and AI to identify markers for cancer early detection.

Adopting the Galleri MCED Test: Personal Experience

The Galleri MCED test, developed by Grail, is not yet FDA-approved and is currently recommended for adults at elevated risk for cancer, such as those aged 50 or older, as a Laboratory Developed Test (LDT). MCED shows significant promise in addressing unmet clinical and public health needs by detecting cancers without existing screening tests. Grail's clinical laboratory is certified under the Clinical Laboratory Improvement Amendments (CLIA) and accredited by the College of American Pathologists, ensuring the Galleri test's clinical utility.

According to Grail's website, the Galleri test does not detect all cancers and should complement routine screening tests recommended by healthcare providers. Results should be interpreted by a healthcare provider within the context of the patient's medical history, clinical signs, and symptoms:

A "Cancer Signal Not Detected" result does not conclusively rule out cancer.

A "Cancer Signal Detected" result necessitates further confirmatory diagnostic evaluations, such as imaging, to confirm cancer. If further testing does not confirm cancer, it may indicate that the cancer is either not present or the test could not detect it, possibly due to its location.

ctDNA Tests for Early Cancer Detection

Pros:

- **Comprehensive Detection: A single blood test can identify over 50 types of cancer, including those lacking screening tests.**
- **Early Detection: Enables the detection of cancer at potentially curable early stages.**
- **High Specificity: Demonstrated specificity of over 99% in multiple large-scale clinical trials, minimizing false positives, unnecessary follow-up tests, and mental stress.**
- **Targeting Aggressive Tumors: Preferentially identifies aggressive tumors, reducing overdiagnosis and overtreatment.**
- **Convenient: A single blood draw without pre-test preparation**

Cons:

- **False Positives and Negatives:**
    - **Unnecessary Follow-up Tests, Mental Stress**
    - **False Sense of Security with Potentially Undetected Tumors**
- **Overdiagnosis and Overtreatment, Particularly for Certain Cancer Types Such As Thyroid and Prostate Cancer**
- **Cost Not Yet Widely Covered by Insurance**
- **Not Yet FDA Approved for Marketing**

After prudently weighing the pros and cons of blood MCED ctDNA tests outlined in the accompanying text box, I felt the benefits clearly outweighed the pitfalls. Thus, I decided to take the Galleri MCED test.

After submitting an online form for the Galleri test, completing a telemedicine consultation and paying for $949, a blood collection kit promptly arrived at my doorstep. I then visited a nearby clinical lab partnered with Grail for the blood draw, which required no fasting or special preparation. The lab then shipped my samples to Grail's facility. A week later, I received an email with my test results. The entire process was smooth and left me with a positive impression.

Here is my MCED test result:

RESULTS SUMMARY

Your result

Galleri®: No Cancer Signal Detected

The Galleri® test did not find any signs of cancer in your blood sample at this time.

It is very important to remember that this test is not able to detect all cancers. Therefore, you should continue to have regular cancer screenings as recommended by your healthcare professional, such as mammograms for breast cancer and colonoscopies for colon cancer.

Acknowledging the straightforwardness and potential impact of the Galleri MCED test, I have incorporated it into my annual health routine. This proactive approach to early screening could significantly enhance my chances of detecting cancer in its earliest stages when treatment is most effective. The convenience and potentially life-saving benefits of this test make it an invaluable part of my preventive healthcare strategy—an investment in peace of mind through early detection.

Experience of MCED Tests by Others

A story illustrating the immense effect of such a screening tool is that of **Roger Royse**. Roger's life turned unexpectedly during a routine flight from Silicon Valley. As he idly flipped through a book on precision medicine, an article about the Galleri blood MCED test, capable of detecting multiple types of cancer early, caught his eye. Intrigued, Roger decided to take the test, never anticipating its profound impact.

In July 2022, Roger received a positive test result and a sobering diagnosis after followup examinations: Stage 2B pancreatic cancer. "Nothing prepares you for those words," Roger recalled. "In an instant, my entire world shifted, and cancer became my sole focus." A conversation with a radiologist revealed just how fortunate Roger's discovery was. "When the radiologist called, he told me I was the luckiest person he'd ever met," Roger recounted. "Given the location and growth of the cancer, I would never have had symptoms. I would have remained unaware until reaching a much more advanced stage. I owe my life to multicancer early-detection testing," he added. Now, Roger is dedicated to living a healthy lifestyle.

Consider **Michael Keller**, a 58-year-old software engineer from San Francisco, who was more preoccupied with debugging code than battling cancer. When he joined the PATHFINDER study and took the Galleri test, it unveiled a hidden threat—early-stage pancreatic cancer. Pancreatic cancer is notoriously stealthy, often striking undetected until it's too late. But this time was different. Thanks to Galleri's MCED, Michael's cancer was caught early. He quickly underwent surgery, and today, he is not just a survivor; he is in remission with a bright future.

Meanwhile, in the heart of Texas, **Laura Stevens** faced her battle. At 62, the retired teacher from Austin was all too familiar with cancer's shadow; it haunted her family history. Determined to change her fate, Laura turned to the Galleri test. The results were startling—bile duct cancer, a rare and aggressive adversary that usually remains hidden until it's too late. But not for Laura. Armed with this early detection, she courageously underwent surgery. Today, her prognosis is a testament to the power of early detection.

In Mile-High City, **Tom Johnson's** story unfolded. At 55, this Denver real estate agent was following his routine health check-up when he decided to include the Galleri test. Little did he know this choice would be transformative. The test identified early-stage small intestine cancer—a diagnosis as rare as finding a diamond in your backyard. Typically, this type of cancer remains undetected until it's advanced. But for Tom, early detection led to surgery, and now he's embracing a healthy future.

Roger, Michael, Laura, and Tom—each faces unique challenges, yet they share a powerful ally: the MCED test. Their experiences transcend medical diagnoses, serving as poignant reminders of the critical importance of early cancer detection. In the battle against cancer, time is invaluable, and early diagnosis significantly enhances the likelihood of successful treatment.

Consider Michael's struggle with pancreatic cancer, Laura's fight against bile duct cancer, and Tom's battle with small intestine cancer. These are among the most elusive cancers, often remaining undetected until it's too late. The MCED test is reshaping this narrative by identifying these silent threats early, at their most curable stage.

These narratives showcase the transformative potential of the MCED test. This blood-based ctDNA test paves the way for early, potentially life-saving interventions by detecting cancers that typically lack other screening methods. The stories of Roger, Michael, Laura, and Tom are not just inspirational—they emphasize the urgent need to incorporate advanced early detection tools like the MCED test into regular preventive healthcare.

Circulating Tumor Cell Tests

Beyond MCED ctDNA tests, circulating tumor cell (CTC) tests present promising opportunities for cancer detection, diagnosis, and management. The concept of circulating tumor cells emerged in the mid-19th century when Australian scientist Thomas Ashworth first identified tumor cells in a cancer patient's blood. However, it was not until the late 20th and early 21st centuries that technological advancements allowed for the detection and analysis of these cells. The development of CTC tests began in the 1990s with the rise of advanced molecular biology techniques, focusing on isolating, counting, and analyzing tumor cells shed from primary or metastatic tumors into the bloodstream.

Today, CTC tests are predominantly utilized in clinical settings for predictive purposes, helping to predict treatment outcomes and monitor disease progression. Over the years, innovations in microfluidics, imaging technologies, and molecular biology have improved the accuracy and efficiency of these tests.

CTC tests have received FDA approval for clinical use, the most notable being the CellSearch system. Approved in 2004, CellSearch is specifically designed to detect and enumerate CTCs in the blood of patients with metastatic breast, prostate, and colorectal cancers, making it the only FDA-approved CTC test for predictive use in these cancers.

Nevertheless, CTC detection tests encounter considerable limitations that hinder their effectiveness, particularly regarding early detection and consistent monitoring. These tests often struggle with low sensitivity and specificity, especially for early-stage cancers where CTCs are scarce, which can result in false negatives. The technical challenges of isolating these rare cells necessitate sophisticated and expensive technologies. Additionally, the lack of standardization across various laboratories and platforms contributes to variability in test results. Furthermore, the biological diversity of CTCs may mean they do not fully represent the characteristics of the primary tumor.

Recently, a novel method has been developed to detect CTCs with enhanced specificity and sensitivity using a chimeric virus probe. This method uniquely identifies live CTCs unaffected by epithelial cell adhesion molecule expression variations. The chimeric virus probe combines a capsid from human papillomavirus for high specificity with an SV40-based genome that amplifies extensively within CTCs, enhancing sensitivity. These innovative features are expected to improve the validity and utility of this CTC detection method.

While CTC tests are primarily employed for monitoring and prognosis in metastatic cancer, ongoing advancements suggest potential applications in early detection. CTC technologies' continued development and refinement are needed to realize their potential in early cancer detection.

The Future of ctDNA Tests in Systemic Early Detection

The cancer screening and early detection field is rapidly evolving, thanks to technological advancements. Innovations like MCED ctDNA tests are set to revolutionize early cancer detection.

Recent technology breakthroughs have greatly improved ctDNA tests. NGS technologies have reduced the cost and time needed for comprehensive genetic analyses, allowing for the detection of trace amounts of tumor DNA in the bloodstream. This facilitates the identification of cancer at its earliest stages. Automation reduces human involvement and enhances efficiency, with systems for sample preparation, DNA extraction, and sequencing managing large volumes of samples with precision. This cuts labor costs and boosts test results' reliability, making ctDNA tests more viable for widespread clinical use.

AI is set to further enhance ctDNA testing by improving the sensitivity and specificity of mutation detection. AI algorithms can analyze vast amounts of genetic data, revealing patterns and biomarkers that may not be obvious to humans. This capability enables more accurate cancer detection, even in asymptomatic individuals, and minimizes the need for repeat testing, improving cost-effectiveness. Additionally, AI can help interpret complex genetic data, providing oncologists with actionable insights for personalized treatment. This integration supports the trend toward precision medicine, where treatments are tailored to each patient's unique genetic profile.

As the use of ctDNA tests increases, economies of scale will help lower costs. A larger user base spreads fixed research, development, and infrastructure expenses across more tests, reducing the expense per test. Moreover, as more healthcare providers adopt ctDNA tests, rising demand will drive further innovations in production and delivery. This scaling effect will make ctDNA tests more accessible to a broader population, including those in underserved areas, helping to reduce healthcare disparities.

In summary, the future of blood MCED ctDNA tests is promising for early cancer detection. Advances in technology, automation, AI integration, and economies of scale will enhance these tests' accuracy, efficiency, and affordability. Consequently, ctDNA tests will become an essential tool in the systemic screening of most cancer types with a single test, ultimately saving lives and reducing the burden and costs of cancer care.

While I have no financial interests in these ctDNA test companies, I am deeply enthusiastic about their potential for proactive, systemic early cancer detection in asymptomatic individuals. This proactive screening approach will transition us from the ineffective symptom-triggered diagnosis and treatment model to an effective early detection and intervention paradigm, minimizing suffering and saving lives.

Given the current dismal outcomes of advanced cancer treatment, prevention, and screening in general, the path to timely regulatory approval and prompt adoption of these innovative MCED tests will be deliberated in the following chapters

.

CHAPTER SEVEN

Unveiling the Black Box of the Human Body

"It was eerie. I saw myself in that machine."
Isidor I Rabi

"Early detection offers the best chance of cure. If you wait for symptoms, you've waited too long. Knowledge is power, and the sooner you have the information, the better".
Robert H. Shmerling, MD

Beyond circulating tumor DNA (ctDNA) tests, is there another tool that can effectively screen for and catch most cancer types early?

In the relentless quest to unveil cancer's insidious presence before it can firmly take root, the advent of ctDNA tests has ushered in a new era of hope. These vanguards of modern medicine, particularly the pioneering Galleri MCED test, promise to detect the faintest whispers of malignancy through a simple blood draw, heralding a paradigm shift in systemic early detection for most cancer types with a single blood test.

However, even as this innovation has captivated the medical community, a sobering reality remains. While the Galleri MCED test boasts an impressive overall sensitivity of 51.5% across all cancer stages, its true strength lies in revealing advanced stages of the disease—attaining a staggering >90% detection rate for stage IV cancers and a formidable 77% for stage III (Galleri, 2021). However, only 16.80% of stage I cancers and 40.40% of stage II cancers are detected, leaving a significant portion of early-stage malignancies undetected. This limitation is clearly linked to the minuscule amount of tumor DNA from early-stage cancers shed into the bloodstream, although current detection sensitivity can be technically improved.

It is in the early stages—those critical windows of opportunity where timely intervention can mean the difference between life and death. As revolutionary as ctDNA tests are, a secondary, systemic early detection method is necessary—a complementary force to maximize the potential of systemic early detection and intervention.

With resolve in scientific exploration, I embarked on a comprehensive review of emerging frontiers in early cancer detection. Among the myriad contenders, one approach stood out—a beacon of promise: **whole-body MRI.**

MRI in Medical Diagnostics

Magnetic Resonance Imaging (MRI) has emerged as a powerful modality in medical diagnostics, offering unparalleled insights into the body's intricate structures and functions. This non-invasive technique has transformed how healthcare professionals approach diagnosis, treatment planning, and monitoring of various medical conditions.

At the heart of MRI lies a potent combination of magnetic fields, radio waves, and advanced computer technology. Unlike X-ray-based imaging, which relies on ionizing radiation, MRI harnesses the principles of nuclear magnetic resonance to generate detailed, high-resolution images of internal organs, tissues, and structures. One of the most remarkable features of MRI is its ability to deliver exceptional soft tissue contrast, enabling precise delineation of anatomical details that would be difficult to visualize with other imaging modalities. This capability has proven invaluable in diagnosing and evaluating various conditions. MRI has proven indispensable in diagnosing and staging cancers, allowing healthcare professionals to detect and characterize tumors at an early stage when treatment is most effective. Using contrast agents, such as gadolinium, enhances the diagnostic capabilities of MRI, providing better visualization of blood vessels, inflammation, and other pathological processes.

In neurological disorders, MRI has revolutionized the diagnosis and management of conditions such as brain tumors, stroke, multiple sclerosis, and neurodegenerative diseases. Its ability to visualize the intricate structures of the brain and spinal cord, combined with advanced techniques like functional MRI, has illuminated the complex workings of the nervous system, aiding in the development of targeted treatments and surgical interventions.

Hence, MRI has emerged as a transformative force in medical diagnostics, offering unparalleled insights into the intricate structures and functions of the human body. Its non-invasive nature, exceptional soft tissue contrast, and ability to visualize a wide range of pathologies have made it an indispensable tool in the diagnosis, treatment planning, and monitoring of various medical conditions. As technology continues to evolve, the future of MRI in medical diagnostics holds immense potential, promising to unlock new frontiers in early detection, patient care, and scientific discovery.

Let's take a moment to explore the evolution of MRI technology and its potential for systemic early cancer detection.

MRI Technology Development

MRI technology is a monumental medical imaging achievement, providing detailed images of the body's internal structures without harmful ionizing radiation. The journey of MRI technology development is a captivating tale of human ingenuity and the relentless pursuit of medical advancement. It began with a simple yet profound question: how can we peer into the human body's inner workings without the harmful effects of radiation?

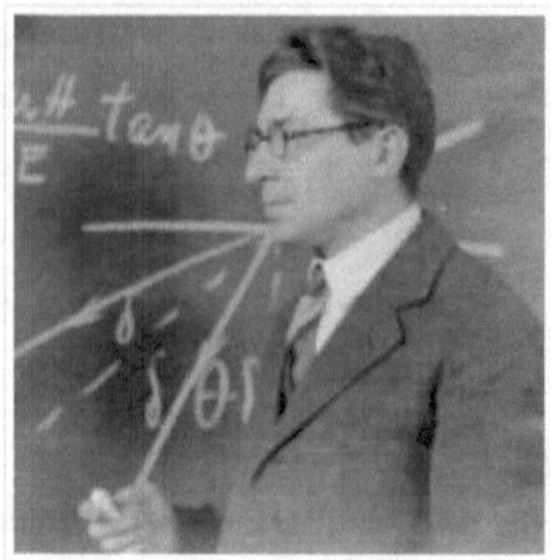

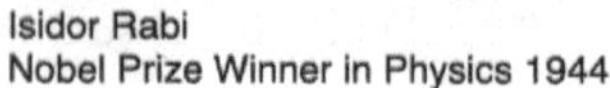

Isidor Rabi
Nobel Prize Winner in Physics 1944

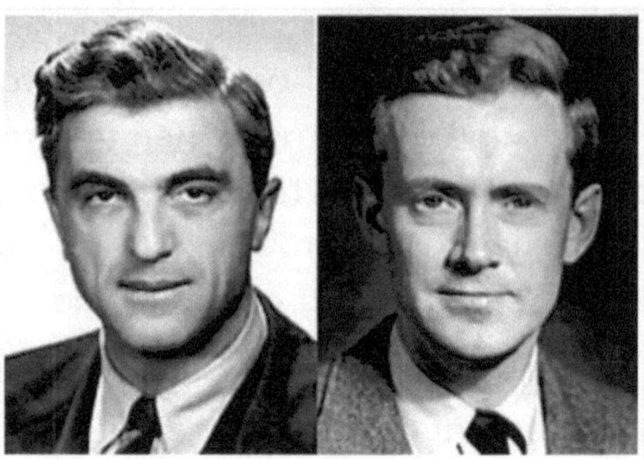

Felix Bloch & Edward Purcell
Nobel Prize Winners in Physics in 1952

The answer lay within theoretical physics, where pioneers like Isidor Rabi, Felix Bloch, and Edward Purcell unraveled the mysteries of nuclear magnetic resonance (NMR). Isidor Rabi, who received the Nobel Prize in Physics in 1944, is credited with discovering NMR. Working at Columbia University in New York City during the 1930s, Rabi and his team measured the magnetic properties of various nuclei, including hydrogen, deuterium, and lithium. Rabi first described how nuclei could flip their magnetic orientation under the influence of an oscillating magnetic field.

Though Rabi is generally credited with discovering NMR, his research was conducted in an "unnatural" context, using a molecular beam in a vacuum to isolate individual nuclei from their environment. It was not until 1945 that independent teams led by Felix Bloch at Stanford and Edward Purcell at MIT simultaneously demonstrated NMR in condensed matter like water. Their discovery, published in the January 1946 issue of Physical Review, showed that atomic nuclei could absorb and emit electromagnetic radiation in a magnetic field. Bloch and Purcell jointly received the Nobel Prize in Physics in 1952 for this and their subsequent work.

Raymond Damadian's 1971 discovery that MRI could distinguish between healthy and cancerous tissues marked a turning point. This led to the creation of the first MRI scanner, "Indomitable," and the first full-body scan in 1977. Paul Lauterbur and Peter Mansfield were instrumental in transforming MRI from a novel concept to a practical diagnostic tool. Lauterbur, at the University of Illinois at Urbana-Champaign, discovered how to create a two-dimensional image by introducing gradients in the magnetic field. At the University of Nottingham, Mansfield refined the use of these gradients. Both were awarded the Nobel Prize in Physiology or Medicine in 2003 for their contributions.

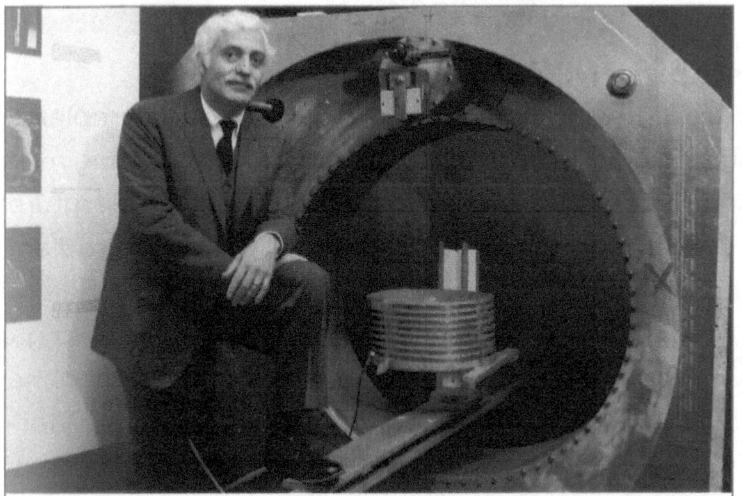

Dr. Raymond Damadian created the first MRI scanner, "Indomitable," and performed the first full-body scan in 1977, now on display in the Hall of Medical Sciences at the Smithsonian Institution.

The commercial development and early adoption of MRI in the 1980s marked a new era in medical diagnostics. Ongoing advancements, such as higher field strengths and specialized techniques like diffusion MRI, further expanded its applications.

The evolution of MRI technology, especially whole-body MRI scanning, represents a significant leap forward. Driven by advancements in hardware and software—such as enhanced image quality, reduced scan times, and AI integration—whole-body MRI has become a comprehensive tool for detecting many conditions, including cancer, across the entire human body.

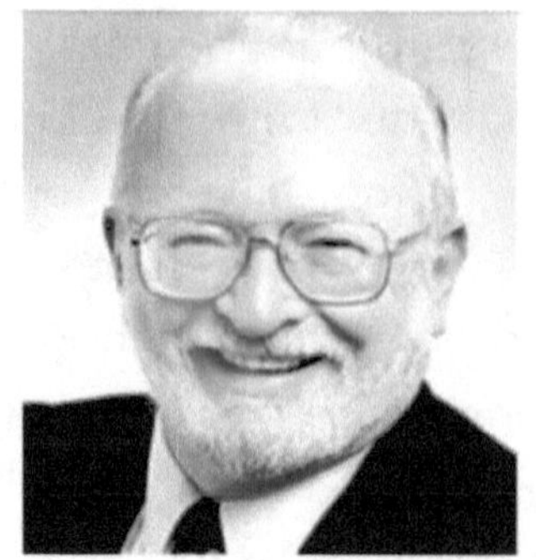

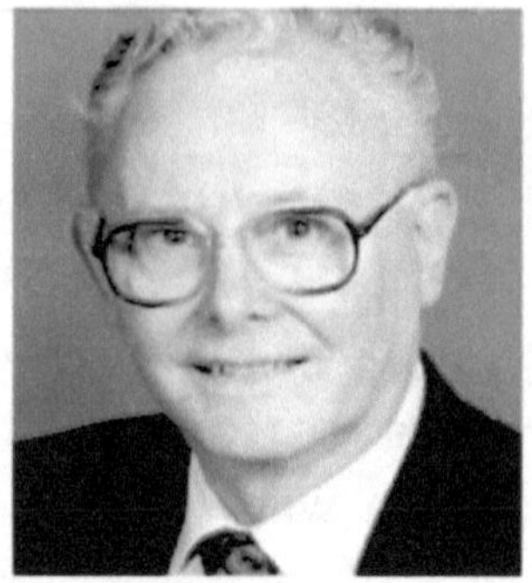

Paul Lauterbur   **Peter Mansfield**
Nobel Prize in Physiology or Medicine 2003

Landscape of MRI Manufacturers

Manufacturing MRI scanners is an intricate and complex process, demanding precise engineering. The superconducting magnets in MRI scanners must be cooled to extremely low temperatures using liquid helium to achieve superconductivity. Gradient coils, essential for spatial encoding of MRI signals, must be crafted to exact specifications to ensure accurate magnetic field gradients and withstand rapid switching, generating substantial heat and mechanical stress. Radiofrequency (RF) systems for signal transmission and reception require highly sensitive and noise-resistant designs, while shielding is necessary to protect against external interference.

Magnetic field strength, measured in Tesla (T) after inventor Nikola Tesla, is crucial for MRI operation. The strength directly impacts the quality and detail of the images produced. High-field MRI scanners (1.5 T to 3.0 T), commonly used in clinical practice, deliver high-resolution images suitable for diagnosing various conditions. For context, the Earth's magnetic field strength is about 50 microteslas (μT), equivalent to 0.00005 Tesla.

Integrating sophisticated software for image reconstruction to enhance diagnostic accuracy adds layers of complexity. Ensuring patient comfort and safety through noise reduction and magnetic shielding, alongside meeting stringent regulatory standards, underscores the multifaceted challenges in MRI scanner manufacturing. This technical endeavor demands a multidisciplinary approach, combining physics, engineering, computer science, and materials science to produce reliable, high-quality MRI systems. Here are the major manufacturers of MRI scanners:

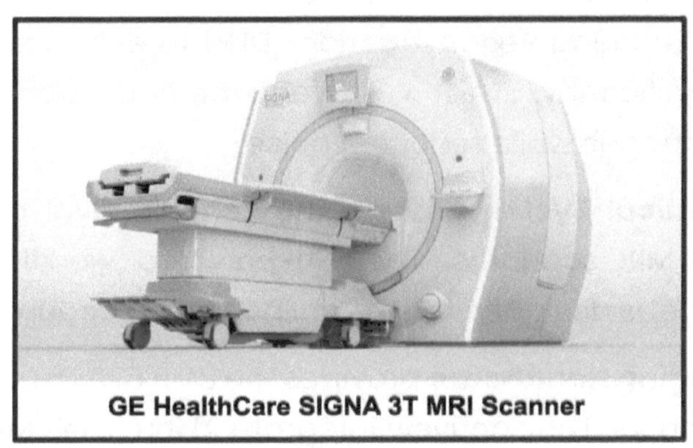
GE HealthCare SIGNA 3T MRI Scanner

GE Healthcare features the SIGNA Premier (3T MRI) and SIGNA Voyager (1.5T MRI) scanners. Their AIR™ Recon DL, a deep learning-based reconstruction technology, significantly enhances image clarity while reducing noise and artifacts. This AI-powered tool ensures faster scans and improved diagnostic confidence, making MRI more efficient and effective.

Siemens Healthineers offers the MAGNETOM Lumina (3T MRI) and MAGNETOM Altea (1.5T MRI) scanners. Siemens integrates AI through its AI-Rad Companion, an AI-powered software suite that assists radiologists by automatically detecting and characterizing abnormalities. Applications like Deep Resolve enhance image quality and reduce scan times, boosting diagnostic accuracy and patient throughput.

Philips Healthcare provides the Ingenia Elition X (3T MRI) and Ingenia Ambition X (1.5T MRI) scanners. Philips' Compressed SENSE technology uses AI to accelerate MRI scans without compromising image quality. This technology cuts scan times by up to 50%, improving patient comfort and throughput. Their AI-powered

IntelliSpace Portal offers advanced visualization and analysis tools to aid radiologists in diagnosis and treatment planning.

Canon Medical Systems (formerly Toshiba Medical Systems) offers the Vantage Galan 3T and Vantage Orian 1.5T MRI scanners. Canon's Advanced Intelligent Clear-IQ Engine (AiCE) technology uses Deep Learning Reconstruction (DLR) to enhance MRI image quality significantly. This AI-driven method produces high-resolution images while reducing noise.

Hitachi Medical Systems offers the Echelon Oval and Echelon Smart 1.5T MRI scanners. Their AI-powered workflow solution, SynergyDrive, is designed to streamline MRI procedures.

United Imaging Healthcare provides the uMR 570 1.5T and uMR 770 3T MRI scanners. They actively integrate AI into their MRI scanners to enhance capabilities and performance.

Neusoft Medical Systems offers the NeuMR 1.5T, SuperMark 1.5T, and NeuMR 0.5T scanners. By incorporating AI into their MRI technology, Neusoft enhances diagnostic accuracy, efficiency, and patient care. For instance, their AI-driven software solutions automatically analyze MRI images to detect anomalies and provide quantitative assessments.

Advantages of MRI over CT

MRI and Computed Tomography (CT) scans are revolutionary diagnostic imaging modalities. While both provide invaluable insights into the human body, MRI offers several advantages over CT scans, making it the preferred choice in various clinical scenarios.

One of the most significant advantages of MRI is its safety, as it does not involve harmful ionizing radiation. In contrast, CT scans utilize X-rays, which can increase the risk of radiation exposure, especially with repeated examinations. This makes MRI the preferred option for whole-body imaging, as it eliminates the potential risks associated with ionizing radiation.

Another notable advantage of MRI is its ability to provide exceptional soft tissue contrast and detail. Unlike CT scans, which rely primarily on density differences to generate images, MRI leverages the magnetic properties of hydrogen atoms in the body to create highly detailed images of soft tissues, such as the brain, spinal cord, muscles, and internal organs. This superior soft tissue contrast makes MRI indispensable for evaluating neurological disorders, musculoskeletal injuries, and pathologies affecting organs like the liver, kidneys, and heart.

MRI also offers unparalleled versatility in imaging planes and sequences. While CT scans primarily provide cross-sectional images, MRI can generate images in any desired plane (axial, sagittal, coronal) without physically moving the patient. This flexibility allows for a comprehensive evaluation of anatomical structures from multiple angles, enhancing diagnostic accuracy and facilitating treatment planning.

Furthermore, MRI boasts the unique capability of functional imaging, such as functional MRI (fMRI), enabling the visualization of brain activity and neurological function mapping. This advanced technique has revolutionized neuroscience, offering invaluable insights into cognitive processes, emotions, and behavior while aiding in diagnosing and managing neurological disorders.

While CT scans excel at imaging bones and detecting fractures, MRI provides superior visualization of soft tissue structures, making it the preferred method for evaluating joint injuries, ligament and tendon tears, and other musculoskeletal conditions. Moreover, MRI offers critical insights into tissue composition and metabolic activity, facilitating early detection and characterization of tumors and other pathologies.

MRI's exceptional soft tissue contrast, non-radiative properties, versatility in imaging planes, and functional imaging capabilities make it indispensable across various medical specialties, including oncology, neurology, orthopedics, and cardiovascular medicine.

MRI Advantage for Whole-Body Scans

Criterion	MRI	CT
Radiation Exposure	No harmful ionizing radiation	Uses harmful ionizing radiation
Soft Tissue Contrast	Superior soft tissue contrast	Inferior soft tissue contrast
Imaging Detail	High detail in soft tissues	Better for bone and lung detail
Safety for Repeated Use	Safe for multiple scans	Risk of cumulative radiation exposure
Versatility	Excellent for brain, muscles, heart, and cancer	Better for detecting bone fractures

MRI Resolution

In modern medicine, the MRI machine serves as a magical looking glass, unveiling the hidden landscapes within our bodies, akin to how a magnifying glass reveals the intricate patterns on a butterfly's wing. However, the clarity of this looking glass varies, and its ability to discern delicate structures beneath our skin depends on MRI resolution.

Imagine a sprawling city viewed from above: from a distance, it's a blur of lights and shadows, but as you descend, individual buildings, streets, and even people come into focus. This is how resolution works in MRI—the power to distinguish between two nearby points, seeing them as distinct entities rather than a merged blur. In our city analogy, it's the difference between perceiving a city block as a single mass or a collection of individual buildings.

Now, envision painting this city on a canvas. The more pixels you use, the more detail you capture. Similarly, in MRI, resolution is tied to the number of voxels (3D pixels) within the Field of View (FOV). More voxels mean higher resolution, just as more brushstrokes create a more detailed painting.

The MRI machine is not just a static device; it's a dynamic character shaped by several factors. The resolution of an MRI scan, defined as the smallest distance between two points that can be differentiated as separate entities, is crucial for image clarity and usefulness. Resolution is directly proportional to pixel count—a greater pixel count results in higher resolution. The resolution of an MRI image is influenced by factors such as magnetic field strength, gradient system, and imaging sequence parameters. There are two types of resolution in MRI: spatial resolution and temporal resolution.

Spatial resolution refers to how small the elements of the image (voxels) are; finer resolution means smaller voxels and more detail. Temporal resolution, essential for dynamic studies like the heart, refers to how quickly images can be acquired. The factors affecting MRI resolution include:

- **Magnetic Field Strength:** Measured in Tesla, this is one of the most significant factors affecting MRI resolution. Higher field strengths provide a higher signal-to-noise ratio, which can be traded off to increase resolution without losing image quality.

- **Gradient System:** The gradient system encodes spatial information and contributes to image sharpness. More powerful gradients with faster switching capabilities allow for finer spatial resolution.

- **Radiofrequency Coils:** The design and capability of the radiofrequency coils (RF coils), which broadcast the RF signal to the patient and receive the return signal, also influence resolution. More sensitive coils can detect finer differences in the magnetic fields of different tissues.

- **Imaging Parameters:** Parameters such as voxel size, matrix size, and the number of acquisitions affect resolution.

Smaller voxels provide higher spatial resolution, while larger matrix sizes capture finer detail.

1.5T and 3T MRI machines are common choices in clinical settings, each offering distinct advantages. Generally, 3T machines provide higher-resolution images due to their stronger magnetic field and increased signal-to-noise ratio (SNR). The choice between these field strengths often hinges on specific clinical requirements and the trade-offs between image quality, scan time, and cost.

1.5T MRI machines are widely favored for balancing cost, safety, and image quality. Typically, they achieve a spatial resolution of about 1-2 mm in-plane (xy-axis) and 2-6 mm through-plane (z-axis), sufficient for most clinical applications. Conversely, 3T MRI machines, with their stronger magnetic fields, generally offer a higher SNR, enabling better spatial resolution or faster imaging times. Under optimal conditions, their spatial resolution can be as fine as 0.5-1 mm in-plane and 1-2 mm through-plane. This makes 3T machines particularly valuable for advanced neuroimaging, functional MRI (fMRI), and small-structure imaging, like visualizing joint cartilage.

Choosing between a 1.5T and a 3T MRI machine involves more than just assessing power. While 3T machines offer finer detail, they can be more prone to artifacts and require additional safety precautions. They are also more expensive. It's a classic trade-off between power and practicality, where clinical needs and resources must be carefully considered.

The evolution of MRI resolution does not stop here. Future advancements in MRI technology, such as improved gradient systems, better RF coil designs, and more sophisticated imaging sequences, promise to push resolution limits even further.

In summary, MRI scans capable of achieving a resolution of 1 mm or smaller can detect tiny cancerous lesions at early, curable stages. The remaining challenge lies in deploying this

technology for early cancer detection in a reliable, efficient, and cost-effective manner.

MRI Sequences and Protocols for Different Body Parts

Now, let's take a closer look at how MRI captures images of various body areas in practice.

MRI harnesses the magnetic properties of atomic nuclei to deliver high-resolution images of soft tissues on the principle of nuclear magnetic resonance. Since the human body is mainly composed of water, the hydrogen nuclei in water molecules are primarily targeted for imaging. When subjected to a magnetic field, these nuclei align with it. A radiofrequency pulse is then applied to disturb this alignment, and as the pulse is turned off, the nuclei revert to their original state, emitting signals in the process. These signals are captured to construct detailed images of the body's internal structures.

MRI Sequence

An MRI sequence refers to the specific settings and parameters used during a scan, which dictate how the signal is acquired and processed to create images. Different tissues require unique MRI sequences due to their distinct properties and how they interact with magnetic fields and radiofrequency pulses. The variation in water, fat, and other tissue components influences their relaxation times ($T1$ and $T2$), necessitating specific sequences for optimal contrast.

For example, T1-weighted sequences highlight structures like the brain's white matter by contrasting fat and water. In comparison, T2-weighted sequences excel at visualizing fluids and edema, making the water appear bright. Some sequences offer higher resolution and anatomical detail, essential for identifying fine structures, such as those in blood vessels and hemorrhages. Specific MRI sequences are also designed to detect particular pathologies and functional changes. Tailoring MRI sequences to tissue-specific properties and clinical needs enhances detection precision.

Each sequence is crafted to spotlight different tissue characteristics and pathologies. Here are some common MRI sequences and their applications:

- **T1-Weighted Sequences (T1W):** These sequences produce images where fat appears bright and water appears dark, using short repetition times (TR) and short echo times (TE). T1W images are excellent for evaluating the anatomy of the brain, distinguishing between grey and white matter, and assessing musculoskeletal structures. They are also used post-contrast to evaluate the vascularity of lesions and the integrity of the blood-brain barrier.

- **T2-Weighted Sequences (T2W):** In these sequences, water appears bright while fat is relatively less bright, achieved through long TR and TE times. T2W images are particularly useful for detecting edema, inflammation, and fluid-filled lesions. They are widely used in brain imaging to detect white matter lesions, spinal imaging to assess disc herniations, and musculoskeletal imaging to identify joint effusions.

- **Diffusion-Weighted Imaging (DWI):** This sequence measures the diffusion of water molecules in tissues, where areas with restricted diffusion appear bright. DWI is crucial for detecting and characterizing tumors, abscesses, and cerebral infarction early. It has emerged as a valuable tool in oncology for tumor detection and characterization since malignant tumors typically exhibit lower apparent diffusion coefficient (ADC) values than surrounding normal tissues, edema, and benign tumors. This is due to the higher cellularity and restricted diffusion of water molecules within malignant lesions. DWI is particularly effective in identifying small tumor foci within the abdomen or peritoneum that may be challenging to detect with conventional imaging methods. DWI can provide essential information for tumor characterization. DWI with background suppression, also known as DWIBS, further enhances the detection of tumors throughout the body by highlighting areas of restricted diffusion.

- **Fluid-Attenuated Inversion Recovery (FLAIR):** FLAIR sequences are a variation of T2W imaging, where a specific inversion pulse nulls the signal from free water, making fluid appear dark. FLAIR is extremely valuable in brain imaging, especially for detecting lesions near the ventricles and in the periventricular region obscured by CSF in regular T2W images.

The choice of MRI sequence and parameters depends on several factors, including tissue type and pathology.

MRI Protocols

MRI protocols are combinations of various MRI sequences tailored to assess specific body regions or pathological processes optimally. These protocols are blueprints for consistent, high-quality diagnostic imaging and efficient radiology service delivery. They aim to maximize diagnostic quality, ensure consistency in scan quality, and enable efficient and effective radiology service delivery.

Developing an MRI protocol involves a delicate balancing act, considering factors such as the region of interest, suspected pathology, time constraints, and available MRI hardware and software capabilities. Protocols typically consist of sequences, each with specific parameters optimized to highlight different tissue characteristics or pathologies. For example, a brain protocol may include T1-weighted, T2-weighted, FLAIR, and diffusion-weighted sequences to thoroughly assess various brain structures and potential abnormalities. These protocols are regularly reviewed and updated to incorporate advancements in MRI technology and evolving clinical needs, ensuring the delivery of state-of-the-art diagnostic imaging services.

For whole-body MRI, protocols are designed to detect and characterize lesions throughout the body. They often incorporate diffusion-weighted imaging (DWI) sequences, which are sensitive to the restricted diffusion of water molecules within highly cellular environments, such as tumors. DWIBS can highlight areas of restricted diffusion, potentially revealing the presence of tumors or metastases. Additionally, whole-body MRI protocols may include contrast-enhanced sequences to improve lesion detection and characterization. Crafting these protocols requires careful consideration of factors such as scan time, patient comfort, and the need for comprehensive coverage while maintaining diagnostic quality. As technology advances, whole-body MRI protocols offer promising early cancer detection, staging, and treatment monitoring opportunities.

MRI's Ability to Distinguish Benign and Malignant Lesions

MRI is a powerful diagnostic tool extensively used in medical practice to identify and differentiate between benign and malignant lesions. The ability to distinguish these lesions is crucial for cancer detection. The contrast in MRI images primarily depends on the differences in the tissues' relaxation times (T1 and T2), reflecting the physical and chemical environment of water molecules within them. By manipulating these parameters, radiologists can obtain high-resolution images that reveal subtle differences in characteristics between benign and malignant lesions.

Characteristics of Benign vs. Malignant Lesions

Morphological Features:

Benign Lesions:

- Shape: Typically well-defined, smooth, and regular borders, often round or oval.

- Margins: Edges are smooth and well-circumscribed, indicating non-invasive growth.

- Size: Generally grows slowly and may remain stable over time.

Malignant Lesions:

- Shape: Often irregular, lobulated, or spiculated due to its invasive nature.

- Margins: Borders are indistinct, ill-defined, or irregular, indicating invasive and infiltrative growth.

- Size: Can grow rapidly with a progressive increase in size.

Signal Intensity on T1-Weighted and T2-Weighted Images:

Benign Lesions:

- T1-Weighted Images: Typically exhibit low to intermediate signal intensity. Some, like lipomas, may appear hyperintense due to high-fat content.

- T2-Weighted Images: Usually show high signal intensity because of fluid or high-water content.

- Malignant Lesions:

- T1-Weighted Images: Present with low to intermediate signal intensity, similar to benign lesions.

- T2-Weighted Images: Often exhibit heterogeneous high signal intensity, reflecting complex internal structures with areas of necrosis, hemorrhage, or cystic changes.

Diffusion-Weighted Imaging (DWI) and Apparent Diffusion Coefficient (ADC) Mapping:

Malignant lesions often restrict diffusion due to high cellular density and reduced extracellular space, resulting in hyperintensity on DWI and low ADC values.

- Benign Lesions: Typically show less restriction of diffusion, appearing less intense on DWI with higher ADC values.

- Malignant Lesions: Often exhibit high signal intensity on DWI and low ADC values, indicative of restricted diffusion.

Here are common benign lesions that can be identified and differentiated by MRI

- Cysts: Fluid-filled sacs occurring almost anywhere in the body, like the kidneys, liver, or ovaries, usually with clear boundaries and non-aggressive growth.

- Hemangiomas: Benign tumors consisting of blood vessels appear in places like the liver, brain, and spinal cord and are sometimes visible on the skin. They vary in size and blood flow, which MRI captures well.

- Lipomas: Soft masses composed mainly of fat cells, often found under the skin or deeper in the body, typically round or oval with a soft, rubbery consistency.

- Fibroadenomas: Commonly found in the breast, these solid benign tumors comprise glandular and fibrous tissues, usually well-defined, mobile, and painless.

- Bone Lesions: These include osteochondromas (bone growths on the external surface of a bone) or enchondromas (cartilage growths within bones), identifiable by their distinctive MRI appearance.

- Adenomas: Benign tumors of glandular origin, such as those in the thyroid or adrenal glands. They can affect hormone levels and may require monitoring or surgical removal if symptomatic.

The differentiation between benign and malignant lesions using MRI is a complex process requiring meticulous analysis of morphological features, signal intensity patterns, contrast enhancement characteristics, and advanced imaging techniques. By mastering these principles, radiologists can deliver accurate diagnoses, guide appropriate treatment decisions, and enhance patient outcomes. As MRI technology advances, the precision in distinguishing between benign and malignant lesions will continue to improve, further solidifying the role of MRI in medical diagnostics.

In summary, MRI scans, with a resolution capacity as small as 1 mm, have the potential to detect and characterize tumors at the earliest stages when used appropriately.

Whole-Body MRI in Preventive Cancer Screening for Patients with Genetic Predispositions—In Practice

Whole-body MRI has emerged as a potent tool in preventive cancer screening for patients with genetic predispositions throughout the whole body to detect tumors at an early stage without exposing patients to ionizing radiation.

Clinical studies have showcased the efficacy of whole-body MRI in detecting cancers in individuals with genetic predispositions, such as Li-Fraumeni syndrome (LFS), hereditary pheochromocytoma-paraganglioma syndromes, and constitutional mismatch repair deficiency. A meta-analysis by Ballinger et al. revealed a cancer prevalence of 7% among 578 subjects with LFS who underwent baseline staging with whole-body MRI. Furthermore, a prospective observational study by Villani et al. on 89 individuals with LFS showed a significant difference in five-year survival rates between the surveillance group undergoing whole-body MRI (88.8%) and the non-surveillance group (59.6%).

Based on promising study results, several professional organizations now recommend whole-body MRI for cancer screening in individuals with genetic predispositions. The National Comprehensive Cancer Network (NCCN) and the American Association for Cancer Research (AACR) endorse whole-body MRI as the preferred screening technique for managing adult and pediatric patients with LFS. Similarly, the MD Anderson Cancer Center advises annual whole-body MRI for pediatric patients with TP53 germline mutations.

The use of whole-body MRI in preventive cancer screening for high-risk individuals underscores the importance of standardized imaging protocols and centralized image reviews. Research shows that institutions with limited experience in cancer screening benefit from centralized reviews by high-volume centers with expertise in managing genetically predisposed patients. This approach ensures consistent and accurate interpretation of findings, ultimately enhancing patient outcomes.

Whole-body MRI in Preventive Cancer Screening for Asymptomatic Individuals—An Emerging Application

In preventive healthcare, a whisper of promise has taken root—the tantalizing potential of whole-body MRI to unveil the body's secrets before they manifest as malignant forces. The clinical results from studies of whole-body MRI for cancer screening in high-risk populations have sparked a growing interest in using this technology as an adjunct to current limited standard screening tests for the general population. As we navigate the uncharted waters of proactive screening, this technology stands as a beacon, illuminating the path toward a future where early detection and personalized care define modern healthcare.

Whole-body MRI's promise lies in its unparalleled ability to detect cancers in their earliest stages, offering a potential revolution in preventive cancer care. With its unmatched sensitivity and safety profile, this technology presents a comprehensive, non-invasive alternative free from the dangers of ionizing radiation.

Whole-body MRI marks a significant advancement in medical diagnostics, providing hope for early cancer detection and intervention across a spectrum of malignancies. Implementing this technology, especially in the general population, requires careful consideration of logistical and technical challenges. Despite these challenges, the potential benefits are undeniable. As research progresses, whole-body MRI could become a cornerstone of preventive health care, offering a non-invasive, comprehensive tool for early cancer detection. With its extensive anatomical coverage and safety profile, whole-body MRI uniquely detects malignant tumors in organs not targeted by current screening programs.

The exploration of whole-body MRI for cancer screening in asymptomatic individuals is gaining momentum, with an increasing number of studies diving into this domain. A review article assessed the data from several investigations on whole-body MRI's efficacy in detecting cancer among asymptomatic individuals. In studies involving 5,809 participants, about 2.0% (119 individuals) exhibited findings suspecting malignant cancer. Among studies that included follow-up and verification, comprising 3,287 screened subjects, 1.5% were confirmed to have malignant cancers histologically.

A recent retrospective study from 2024 sheds light on whole-body MRI's potential for early cancer detection in asymptomatic individuals. This study, encompassing 2,064 participants, provides robust data to evaluate the technology's effectiveness in a general population. The findings reveal that 43 individuals, or 2.1% of the sample, showed signs suggestive of malignancy. Of these, 24 participants, representing 1.2%, were confirmed to have cancer, indicating a significant detection rate in an asymptomatic cohort. Conversely, 19 individuals received false-positive results, yielding a false-positive rate of approximately 0.9%. The positive predictive value (PPV) was around 55.8%, signifying that over half of the suspicious findings were actual cancers.

While whole-body MRI holds promise in cancer detection with a relatively low false-positive rate, further research is essential to evaluate its long-term benefits, potential pitfalls, and overall cost-effectiveness. A balanced approach is necessary, weighing the advantages of early detection against the risks of overdiagnosis and unnecessary interventions.

Potential Pitfalls of MRI for Early Detection

Adopting whole-body MRI in preventive healthcare has sparked ferocious debate over its efficacy and potential consequences, notably false positives, overdiagnosis, and overtreatment.

As the medical community grapples with these challenges, navigating these concerns responsibly and effectively becomes crucial. Due to the high sensitivity of MRI, issues of false positives and overdiagnosis are particularly pronounced.

Misidentified Benign Lesions—False Positives

False positives in MRI imaging, mainly due to misidentified benign lesions, are a significant concern. A false positive occurs when diagnostic tests incorrectly suggest the presence of a disease, such as cancer when it is not present. This can cause psychological distress, increased healthcare costs, and unnecessary tests that may carry their risks. MRI typically distinguishes these benign lesions from malignant ones due to its ability to provide detailed images based on the different magnetic properties of tissues. However, misidentification of benign lesions as suspicious or indeterminate can still occur.

Artifact Lesions—False Positives

Like all imaging techniques, MRI has its limitations and potential complications. A notable issue is the creation of artifacts, which can mimic or suggest pathological lesions, known as "artifact lesions." Artifacts in MRI are discrepancies between the produced images and the actual anatomical structures. These artifacts can appear in various forms. Motion artifacts are caused by patient movement during the scan. Chemical shift artifacts result from different fat and water resonance frequencies, creating misleading appearances at tissue boundaries. Truncation artifacts, also known as Gibbs artifacts, arise from the finite number of data points used in MRI image reconstruction, leading to ringing effects near sharp edges, which can be mistaken for structural abnormalities. However, the occurrence and impact of artifact lesions can be mitigated with sequence optimization, education and awareness, and technological advances.

Indeterminate Lesions

Despite its sophistication, MRI sometimes cannot definitively characterize certain lesions, rendering them indeterminate. Understanding why some lesions remain ambiguous involves examining the inherent limitations of the technology, the biological complexity of lesions, and patient-specific factors. Here are common reasons for Indeterminate Lesions:

- **Biological Complexity of Lesions:** Benign or malignant lesions often exhibit significant heterogeneity. Different parts of the same lesion may have varying histological and biochemical properties, leading to mixed signal characteristics on MRI. This heterogeneity complicates MRI scan interpretation as radiologists may encounter conflicting information within a single lesion. Some benign and malignant lesions share similar imaging characteristics, making differentiation difficult. For example, both benign fibroadenomas and malignant breast carcinomas can appear as well-circumscribed masses on MRI, and certain liver lesions, such as focal nodular hyperplasia and hepatocellular carcinoma, may exhibit similar enhancement patterns. This overlap necessitates additional diagnostic tools or follow-up imaging for a definitive diagnosis.

- **Inherent Limitations of MRI Technology:** While MRI offers superior resolution to many other imaging modalities, it is still limited by its spatial resolution. Small lesions or those in anatomically complex regions may not be imaged with sufficient detail for definitive characterization. The fine structures within these lesions might be below the resolution threshold, leading to ambiguity. While MRI distinguishes tissues based on differences in their relaxation times (T1 and T2) and proton density, the signal intensity of benign and malignant lesions can overlap significantly, particularly in the early stages of the disease. This overlap makes differentiation challenging, especially when morphological features and signal characteristics are not distinct. Noise in the images can also mask subtle differences between tissues, leading to indeterminate findings.

- **Influence of Patient-Specific Factors:** Variations in patient anatomy can impact the visibility and characterization of lesions. For instance, dense breast tissue in younger women can obscure lesions, making them harder to characterize. Similarly, the proximity of lesions to complex anatomical structures, such as blood vessels or organs, can complicate MRI scan interpretation. Patients with multiple medical conditions or previous treatments, such as surgery or radiation therapy, may have altered tissue characteristics that affect MRI interpretation. Scar tissue, inflammation, or edema can mimic or mask lesions, leading to indeterminate findings.

Indolent Lesions: Overdiagnosis and Overtreatment

In medical terms, "indolent" refers to a condition that remains asymptomatic and non-progressive for an extended period. Indolent lesions are low-risk anomalies with minimal potential for progression. These indolent lesions can be detected by whole-body MRI, resulting in unnecessary and sometimes invasive follow-up procedures that pose risks without providing real benefits to the patient.

Overdiagnosis happens when a medical test identifies a disease or condition that will never cause symptoms or lead to death within a patient's lifetime. Detecting indolent lesions may trigger a cascade of additional tests and unnecessary treatments.

The detection of indolent lesions may result in overtreatment—a situation where the treatment is more aggressive than needed or where no treatment is required at all. Overtreatment can cause various adverse effects, such as unnecessary surgeries or radiation, and their accompanying physical and psychological side effects. For example, a patient diagnosed with a slow-growing tumor might undergo surgery or chemotherapy, both of which carry their risks and complications, potentially diminishing quality of life or even leading to premature mortality.

Active Surveillance—Prostate and Thyroid Cancer Case Studies

Prostate and thyroid cancers exemplify how cancer screening can lead to overdiagnosis and overtreatment. Active surveillance is a management approach used for certain early-detected, low-risk cancers such as prostate and thyroid cancers. Instead of immediate treatment, this approach closely monitors the patient's condition to track cancer progression. It strikes a balance between vigilance and avoiding unnecessary treatments, aiming to maintain the patient's quality of life while ensuring timely medical intervention if the cancer advances. This approach necessitates a strong partnership between the patient and the healthcare team to monitor and respond to changes effectively.

Prostate Cancer: Screening for prostate cancer typically involves measuring prostate-specific antigen (PSA) levels in the blood and MRI imaging. Elevated PSA levels can indicate the presence of prostate cancer, but they can also result from benign conditions such as prostatitis or benign prostatic hyperplasia. The widespread use of PSA testing has led to a dramatic increase in the diagnosis of clinically insignificant tumors that would not have caused symptoms or death.

Treatments for prostate cancer, including surgery and radiation therapy, can lead to significant side effects such as erectile dysfunction, urinary incontinence, and bowel problems. For many men with slow-growing prostate cancers, the side effects of treatment can lead to a decrease in quality of life, potentially outweighing the benefits of treating a cancer that is unlikely to affect their health significantly.

Newer guidelines recommend shared decision-making for PSA screening, where patients and providers consider the potential benefits and harms of screening based on individual risk factors such as age, family history, and patient preferences. Active surveillance is often used for managing patients with prostate cancer.

Thyroid Cancer. The increased use of ultrasonography and medical imaging has notably surged the detection of thyroid cancer, particularly papillary thyroid microcarcinomas, which are very slow-growing. Despite the spike in diagnoses, studies indicate that the mortality rate for thyroid cancer has remained relatively stable, highlighting the issue of overdiagnosis. Typically, thyroid cancer treatment involves surgically removing the thyroid, followed by lifelong thyroid hormone replacement therapy.

Although this surgery is generally safe, it can lead to complications such as damage to the parathyroid glands or vocal cords. The necessity of such treatments for tiny, slow-growing cancers has become increasingly scrutinized within the medical community.

There is a growing advocacy for a conservative approach to managing small papillary thyroid cancers through active surveillance rather than immediate surgery, similar to the watchful waiting strategies employed in prostate cancer.

The concerns of overdiagnosis and overtreatment underscore the need for a balanced approach to cancer screening. This approach should consider the risks and benefits of detecting and treating early-stage cancers. As awareness of these issues rises within the medical community, it is crucial to update screening guidelines and educate patients about the potential outcomes of screening, enabling them to make informed health decisions.

Psychological and Economic Implications

The detection of a lesion by MRI, even when ultimately benign, can cause significant psychological distress. The initial diagnosis of a potentially severe illness can be traumatic, and the emotional turmoil often persists despite a final benign diagnosis. The uncertainty between initial detection and final results can be intense, with long-lasting effects on a patient's mental health.

The psychological impact of false positives and overdiagnosis cannot be overstated. Patients diagnosed with conditions that might never affect their health still endure the emotional and psychological stress of a cancer diagnosis. The associated anxiety, fear, and stress can significantly affect lifestyle and mental health, even if the disease would not have impacted their physical health during their lifetime.

Scanxiety: Research in psychology and oncology has documented "scanxiety," the anxiety linked to medical imaging and the wait for results. This heightened state of stress is unpleasant and can also negatively impact physical health, contributing to increased heart rate, high blood pressure, and a weakened immune response.

Economically, false positives, overdiagnosis, and overtreatment drive up healthcare costs. Unnecessary treatments and follow-up procedures consume resources that could be better allocated to more urgent healthcare needs. Such misallocation implications are particularly severe in systems where healthcare resources are strained.

Ethical Considerations

The ethical implications of whole-body MRI scans for screening and early diagnosis deserve careful thought. Balancing the benefits of early disease detection with the risks of overdiagnosis and overtreatment is complex. Medical ethics dictate that interventions should do more good than harm—a principle challenged by the frequent false positives associated with whole-body MRI.

Detecting indolent lesions through whole-body MRI raises significant ethical questions, particularly the fundamental medical principle of "do no harm." The value of such diagnostic practices must be scrutinized when detecting a lesion that causes more harm than its potential progression.

Criticisms of Preventive Whole-body MRI

Whole-body MRI scans are highly sensitive and can identify various abnormalities. However, given the potential pitfalls, some experts strongly criticize their use for preventive care in asymptomatic individuals.

Dr. Barnett Kramer, former Director of the Division of Cancer Prevention at the National Cancer Institute, has raised concerns about the psychological impact of false positives. He argues that the anxiety and stress caused by unnecessary follow-up tests can outweigh the potential benefits of early cancer detection. Kramer advocates for a balanced screening approach, emphasizing the importance of considering both psychological and physical harms alongside potential benefits.

The medical community has not established specific guidelines for using whole-body MRI in cancer screening. Dr. Rebecca Smith-Bindman, a radiologist and researcher at the University of California, San Francisco, has called for more rigorous standards. She stresses the importance of evidence-based protocols to ensure that imaging techniques, including whole-body MRI, are employed appropriately and effectively.

Dr. Gilbert Welch, a noted critic of overdiagnosis, has pointed out that advanced imaging techniques, like whole-body MRI, can detect benign or indolent lesions that may not require treatment. In his book "Overdiagnosed: Making People Sick in the Pursuit of Health," Welch argues that increased imaging can lead to a cascade of follow-up tests and treatments, potentially causing more harm than good.

Dr. Otis Brawley, former Chief Medical Officer of the American Cancer Society, advocates for evidence-based screening practices. He notes that many cancers detected by whole-body MRI may never cause symptoms or affect patients' lifespans, leading to overdiagnosis and overtreatment. This perspective is reinforced by the absence of large-scale, randomized controlled trials showing a clear benefit of whole-body MRI in cancer screening over standard methods such as mammography, colonoscopy, and low-dose CT scans.

Dr. Welch and Dr. Brawley emphasize prioritizing public health measures that benefit the most people. They argue that focusing on whole-body MRI for cancer screening may divert attention and resources from more equitable and effective public health interventions.

Medical Societies' Stance on Preventive MRI

Medical societies express caution regarding using whole-body MRI for routine cancer screening.

- **American College of Radiology (ACR):** The ACR does not recommend whole-body MRI for cancer screening in asymptomatic individuals due to a lack of evidence supporting its effectiveness and the potential for overdiagnosis and false positives. The ACR advocates the use of established, evidence-based screening methods.

- **U.S. Preventive Services Task Force (USPSTF):** The USPSTF does not recommend whole-body MRI for cancer screening. The task force underscores the need for more research to ascertain the benefits and harms of whole-body MRI compared to traditional screening methods. The USPSTF supports screening practices backed by strong evidence that has been shown to reduce cancer mortality.

While whole-body MRI scans provide a sensitive method for detecting potential health issues, their use for cancer screening and preventive care remains contentious. Critics point out the high costs, risks of overdiagnosis and overtreatment, false positives, lack of specific guidelines, and ethical concerns about resource allocation. As this debate unfolds, it is vital to consider the implications of adopting new preventive care technologies.

To Act or To Wait?

Whole-body MRI holds promise for preventive screening, yet its use in asymptomatic individuals is met with apprehension and uncertainty. No professional medical society in the US currently endorses whole-body MRIs as a proactive screening tool. While early cancer detection can save lives, there is still a lack of sufficient data to demonstrate its effectiveness in reducing cancer deaths in asymptomatic populations.

My primary physician and colleagues have all expressed concerns about the pitfalls, as discussed earlier.

However, being over 50 years old puts me at high risk despite having no symptoms or other risk factors. For a non-smoking male like me, the only recommended cancer screenings are colonoscopy and an optional PSA test. That's it.

I have thoroughly reviewed the relevant literature and information. Here is a summary of the pros and cons of preventive whole-body MRI that I prepared for myself.

Whole-Body MRI Scans for Systemic Early Cancer Detection

Pros:

- **Systemic, Preventive Early Detection Of Cancer:**
    - Identify cancerous lesions throughout the body
    - Currently recommended for individuals with genetic cancer disposition syndromes
- **High Sensitivity: Capable of Identifying Tiny Cancerous Lesions At Curable Early Stages With a Resolution Limit at 1-mm or Smaller**
- **Safe: Without Exposure To Radiation**
- **Painless And No Pre-scan Preparation**
- **No Better Alternative For Systemic Early Cancer Detection**
- **Systemic Detection Of Other Medical Conditions (>500)**

Cons:

- **False Positives And Negatives:**
    - Most lesions identified are benign, potentially causing unnecessary follow-up tests
    - Mental stress
    - False sense of security with potentially undetected tumors
- **Overdiagnosis And Overtreatment, Particularly For Certain Cancer Types, Such As Thyroid And Prostate Cancer**
- **Lack of Randomized Controlled Clinical Trials In General Populations**
- **Not Recommended For General Populations By Medical Societies**
- **Cost Not Covered By Insurance**

After cautiously weighing the pros and cons, I reached a clear conclusion: a definite yes. To me, the benefits of proactive early detection far outweigh the potential risks.

Of course, making a decision or recommendation at a societal level is much more complex. It requires definitive evidence from large, randomized trials, which could be decades away for preventive whole-body MRI, and consideration of many other factors such as broad applicability, equality, and cost-effectiveness.

Landscape of Whole-body MRI Service Providers

Having decided to proceed, I reviewed the landscape of preventive whole-body MRI service providers to select a high-quality option for my scan.

Full-body MRI scans have been available for years but were traditionally very expensive. Recent technological advancements and price reductions have made them much more accessible.

Regulation for Providing Services with Medical Devices

Offering whole-body MRI scans for cancer screening in healthy individuals involves several regulatory requirements to ensure safety, efficacy, and ethical standards. These requirements can vary by country or region. Here is a general overview of the regulatory mandates for companies providing preventive whole-body MRI in healthy persons:

- **Compliance with Medical Device Regulations:** MRI machines are classified as medical devices and must adhere to relevant regulations. In the US, MRI machines must be approved or cleared by the FDA under the 510(k) process or through premarket approval (PMA). In the European Union, MRI machines must comply with the Medical Device Regulation (MDR) and obtain a CE mark, indicating conformity with health, safety, and environmental protection standards.

- **Facility Accreditation:** Imaging centers must be accredited by recognized bodies such as the American College of Radiology (ACR) in the United States or other relevant organizations in their respective regions. Accreditation ensures that the facility meets quality standards in imaging procedures, equipment maintenance, and staff qualifications.

- **Professional Qualifications and Training:** The facility must employ qualified radiologists and technicians trained and certified to perform and interpret MRI scans. Continuous professional education and training are required to maintain certification.

- **Data Privacy and Security:** Compliance with the Health Insurance Portability and Accountability Act (HIPAA) to protect patient data privacy and security.

- **Marketing and Advertising Regulations:** Marketing materials and advertisements must be truthful and not misleading.

Leading Whole-Body MRI Service Providers

An increasing number of full-body MRI scan service providers have emerged. Several trailblazing companies are at the forefront of this preventive whole-body MRI service, each with a unique story, distinctive facilities, and notable accomplishments.

Prenuvo

Prenuvo, co-founded by Andrew Lacy and Dr. Raj Attariwala in 2018, is at the forefront of preventive whole-body MRI. Their mission is to shift the focus of healthcare from reactive "sick" care to proactive preventive care by offering comprehensive scans capable of detecting over 500 conditions, including early-stage cancers and aneurysms. An experienced entrepreneur, Lacy envisioned Prenuvo to make advanced medical imaging accessible to everyone. Despite challenges in merging cutting-edge technology with user-friendly services, the company has emerged as a beacon of hope in early detection and preventive care.

Dr. Attariwala, inspired by a family friend's late-stage cancer diagnosis, developed an AI-powered MRI machine that can scan individuals faster than traditional systems. Prenuvo's non-invasive scans eliminate the need for radiation and contrast dyes, ensuring patient safety while utilizing advanced AI analysis to identify anomalies quickly. These detailed scans provide insights into multiple organs and systems, detecting conditions such as solid tumors, spinal degeneration, and metabolic disorders. Prenuvo's approach has set a new standard for early disease detection and proactive health management.

Supported by prominent figures like Cindy Crawford, Anne Wojcicki, Tony Fadell, and Eric Schmidt and funded by Felicis Ventures, Prenuvo has expanded to multiple locations in the US and Canada, with plans for further growth. Prenuvo advocates for full-body MRIs to be used as a screening tool, akin to colonoscopies or mammograms, to detect early-stage cancer.

Ezra

Emi Gal's vision for Ezra was inspired by a profound desire to democratize cancer screening by integrating advanced MRI technology and artificial intelligence (AI). Originating in New York City, Ezra's journey has been marked by rapid growth and technological advancements, positioning it at the forefront of the AI-driven imaging revolution.

Ezra has integrated AI technology into all three key components of the cancer screening process: imaging, analysis, and reporting. By harnessing AI, Ezra aims to make full-body MRI scans more affordable and accessible. The company has reduced the price of its full-body MRI scan by 40%. Ezra's innovative approach and rapid expansion underscore the growing demand for preventive healthcare solutions. By offering detailed, non-invasive whole-body MRI scans, Ezra aims to establish a new standard of preventive care and empower people with the knowledge to make informed health decisions.

Supported by prominent investors such as Healthier Capital, FirstMark Capital, Allianz Life Ventures, and others, Ezra has secured funding to accelerate its expansion across North America and advance the use of its AI technology.

SimonMed Imaging

SimonMed Imaging is a leading outpatient medical imaging provider founded by Dr. John Simon, a renewed radiologist. SimonMed Imaging operates a large network of outpatient centers across several states in the US, making it convenient for patients to access their services. Each center is equipped with advanced imaging technology and staffed by experienced radiologists and technologists. SimonMed aims to provide high-quality, affordable medical imaging services by leveraging advanced technology and expert radiologists to deliver precise diagnostic results.

SimonOne of SimonMed Imaging provides its preventive whole-body MRI. This service aims to detect potential health issues early, even before symptoms appear. Preventive MRI can screen for various conditions, including cancer, cardiovascular diseases, and neurological disorders, providing patients with peace of mind and the opportunity for early intervention. SimonMed is known for its competitive pricing, which is often lower than hospital-based imaging services. Moreover, SimonMed's SimonOne Imaging services offer a comprehensive suite of imaging modalities, including MRI, CT, Ultrasound, and Mammography. Their preventive MRI services, in particular, provide valuable insights into a patient's health, promoting early detection and intervention.

RadNet

RadNet is a national leader in delivering high-quality, cost-effective diagnostic imaging services through its network of outpatient imaging centers. Offering comprehensive medical imaging, including whole-body MRI, RadNet operates numerous locations across the United States. The company employs advanced MRI machines, such as the 1.5T Wide-Open MRI, 3T Wide-Open MRI, and Open MRI systems. Board-certified radiologists and highly trained technologists ensure the utmost quality and accuracy in imaging and interpretation.

Dr. Berger, a renewed radiologist, co-founded RadNet Inc. in 1980 and has served as its president and CEO. Under his leadership, RadNet has expanded into one of the largest radiology imaging companies in the country, with over 360 outpatient imaging centers in eight states, generating approximately $1.6 billion in revenue last year. The company is also integrating artificial intelligence algorithms across all its imaging centers.

Halo Diagnostics

Founded by experienced radiologists and healthcare entrepreneurs, including Dr. John Feller, Halo Dx represents a fusion of expertise and innovation. The company is dedicated to integrating advanced technology to improve patient outcomes.

Halo Dx offers comprehensive MRI scans that reveal the body's innermost details. From lung screenings to body composition analysis, Halo Dx's optional add-ons provide a personalized approach to preventive care.

BodyView

BodyView, an MRI Scan & Imaging Center division, has led the way in advanced medical diagnostic imaging for the past three decades. In the sunny state of Florida, Dr. Robert L. Kagan set out to advance medical imaging. With over thirty years of experience, Dr. Kagan is a nationally renowned expert in diagnostic imaging. His journey began in 1984 with the introduction of Florida's first

FDA-approved free-standing MRI, allowing for advanced scans outside of a hospital setting. In the 1990s, Dr. Kagan continued to innovate, bringing research-grade high-field MRI scanners from academia to outpatient settings.

Today, with BodyView, Dr. Kagan continues his mission to provide advanced medical imaging services that detect health issues early. Specializing in whole-body MRI scans, BodyView aims to identify life-threatening illnesses like cancer at their earliest stages. The Whole-Body MRI Scan thoroughly examines major organs and systems without the risks associated with ionizing radiation. Dr. Kagan's facility houses the GE Discovery MR 750 3.0 Tesla High Field MRI system, a state-of-the-art device that ensures the highest quality imaging comparable to those found in leading diagnostic and research institutions.

ARISTRA

Meanwhile, across the Atlantic in Germany and Switzerland, ARISTRA emerges as a beacon in medical imaging. Founded by esteemed practitioners, ARISTRA unites specialists from diverse disciplines, infrastructure providers, globally renowned researchers, and patients, all striving for optimal MRI imaging. Michael Ho, MD, leads this distinguished network.

Throughout Germany and Switzerland, ARISTRA's radiologists offer comprehensive MRI scans in partner practices. These scans provide a panoramic view of the body's hidden realms, designed to detect potential health issues early. By offering such advanced imaging, ARISTRA aims to illuminate health concerns before they manifest, fostering early detection and intervention for a healthier future.

Other Companies Offering Preventive Whole-Body MRI Services:

- **Next Health:** Co-founded by Dr. Darshan Shah and Kevin Peake, Next Health provides a range of health optimization services, including full-body MRI scans, in Los Angeles, New York, and Miami.

- **Rezolut:** Rezolut is a national platform specializing in advanced medical imaging technologies, including preventive whole-body MRI, operating in numerous centers across the United States.

- **Smart Heart and Health Preventive Imaging:** Led by renowned radiologist Dr. Bradley A. Jabour in Santa Monica, CA, they offer the ZeroRad Scan, a whole-body MRI for preventive health screening.

- **Full Body Scan Company (London):** Provides comprehensive MRI scans covering the entire body to detect potential health issues before symptoms appear.

These pioneers of preventive whole-body MRI imaging are ushering in a new era of preventive healthcare for early detection and intervention.

Cleveland Clinic, Mayo Clinic, Duke Health, Mount Sinai Health System, Stanford Health Care, and other major medical centers in the US also offer preventive whole-body MRI scans as part of their executive health programs.

My Experience with Prenuvo's Whole-Body MRI

Prenuvo's mission, as stated on their website, resonates with me.
I also greatly appreciate their meticulous efforts in ensuring MRI quality, which is crucial for the accurate early detection of abnormalities. Several factors contribute to the high image quality in Prenuvo's whole-body MRI screening exams, including optimizing voxel size, multi-parametric imaging, and diffusion-weighted imaging (DWI), one of the most critical sequences for early cancer detection.

> ## See today what could happen tomorrow
>
> The current healthcare system is designed to treat illness, not prevent it. But you deserve to know what's going on in your body — even before symptoms appear.
>
> At the heart of our work are thoughtfully designed clinics and cutting-edge optimized MRI hardware and software. Coupled with our AI research and the largest database of whole body imaging in the world, Prenuvo lets you experience the future of proactive health, today.
>
> **Source: Prenuvo**

After reviewing various options, I chose Prenuvo for my whole-body MRI scan and experienced the entire process seamlessly, from online booking to scanning and post-scan consultation.

After setting up an online account and completing the order form, I paid a refundable reservation fee of $2499. While the cost of whole-body MRI scans may seem steep for a middle-class family like mine, it is pretty reasonable compared to other expenses such as airfare, hotel stays, and other leisure activities. I have decided to prioritize health and preventive care above less critical pursuits by reallocating resources for annual preventive care not covered by health insurance for myself and my family.

I scheduled my scan during a lunch break at the modern Prenuvo MRI Center on Wilshire Blvd, Los Angeles, CA, using a customized 1.5T MRI scanner on November 1, 2022. Preparation for MRI scans was minimal, requiring only a four-hour fast. After changing into a gown and removing any metal objects like my iPhone, keys, and watch, I lay on the scanner table and donned earphones to listen to my choice of music. The scan lasted about 60 minutes, with occasional voice prompts to hold my breath for 20 seconds during chest and abdomen scans. The entire procedure was smooth and comfortable.

A week later, I received an email notification that my personalized Prenuvo report was ready. The whole-body MRI images were uploaded to my Prenuvo account for online viewing and download.

In my Prenuvo online account, the face page of the Scan Report displays:

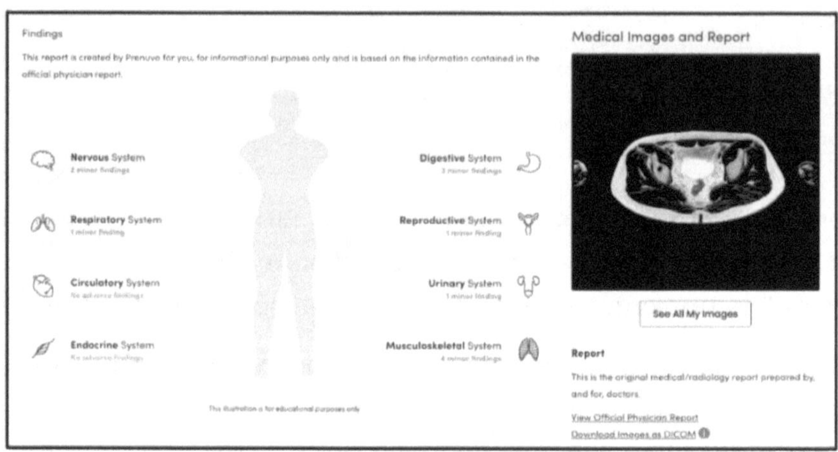

Online Report of My Full-Body MRI Scan (Prenuvo, 2022)

I explored the full online report, which provided comprehensive images of all my internal organs. The report was thorough, detailing every major organ system. Below are some representative images from my whole-body MRI.

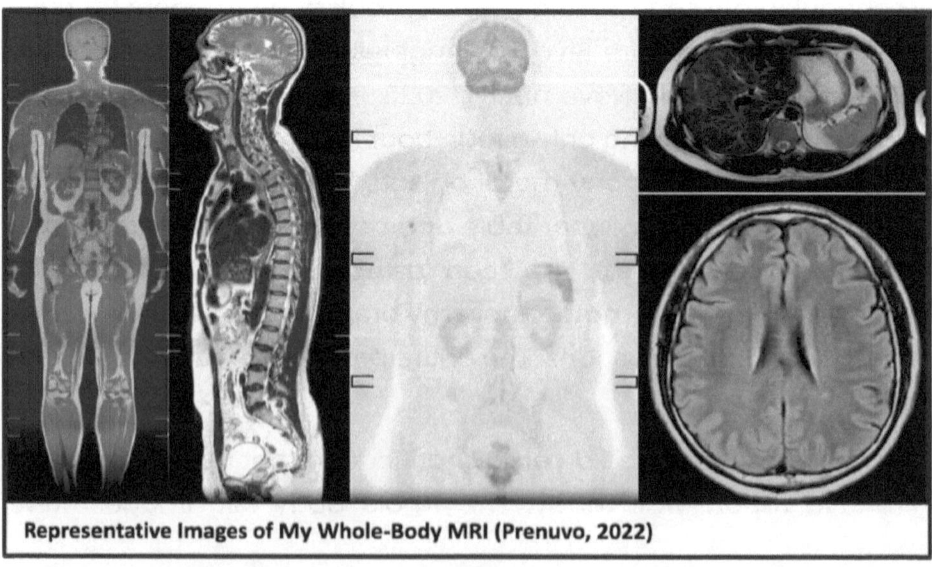

Representative Images of My Whole-Body MRI (Prenuvo, 2022)

Prenuvo sent me a PDF Scan Report via email alongside the online report. This report included a two-page summary featuring Scan Techniques used for various body parts, a Discussion section explaining scan limitations, a Final Impression section listing any detected abnormalities, and a Next Appointment section.

Here are the detailed scan techniques and Discussion section provided in the two-page summary.

> **TECHNIQUE:**
> Head: Flair, TOF, 3DT1; Neck: Axial T2; Whole-body: T1, STIR , DWI; Spine: Sagittal T2; Chest/Abdomen/Pelvis: axial T2; Abdomen: Axial T2, Pelvis: Ax T2 Small FOV, DWI

> **DISCUSSION:**
> The patient was advised that whole-body screening: (i) does not evaluate the heart, (ii) does not evaluate lung microarchitecture, but will assess for mediastinal/hilar adenopathy, (iii) is not a replacement for colonoscopy but will detect bowel carcinoma constricting the colon, (iv) no cartilage based sequences are performed which limits detailed assessment of the joints, and (v) is effective for visualization of lesions on the order of 1 cm or larger within the neck, chest, abdomen and pelvis. As with any medical test, there are limitations which make it impossible to detect all malignancies.

In whole-body MRI, the scanning technique serves as a cartographer's blueprint—a meticulously crafted protocol that reveals the body's intricate tapestry. This imaging modality orchestrates a symphony of sequences, each note resonating with screening potential.

Sequences like FLAIR, TOF, and 3DT1 for the cerebral region provide detailed anatomical insights. In the cervical spine, axial T2 sequences illuminate the neck's complex pathways. The entire body is mapped with the resonant melodies of T1, STIR, and DWI sequences, while the spinal column's sagittal T2 sequence offers a cohesive backdrop.

Axial T2 sequences capture intricate anatomical details in the thoracic and abdominal regions. The pelvic area receives a focused evaluation through axial T2 and DWI sequences.

The MRI Scan Report's Final Impression section reveals several cysts of various sizes in my kidneys and liver. It also notes numerous degenerative changes in my shoulders, spine, knees, ankles, and other parts of the musculoskeletal system, consistent with my age. Additionally, there is mild fat deposition in my liver, and the prostate volume is calculated at 31 mL, slightly above the average of 30 mL or less. Radiologist Stephanie Coleman, MD, signed the MRI Scan Report.

Following the two-page summary, the report includes images of the detected abnormalities and a comprehensive, organ-by-organ analysis.

With relief, no suspicious nodules or lesions were detected in my whole-body MRI.

An online Zoom meeting with a nurse practitioner was scheduled to explain the scan results and answer my questions. In my case, no immediate follow-up scan was necessary. According to the website, Prenuvo's whole-body MRI screening serves as an adjunct to, but does not replace, other established evidence-based screening practices for the early detection of specific malignancies (e.g., colonoscopy, dedicated breast imaging, Pap smear screening for cervical cancer, low-dose chest CT for high-risk patients).

The Pleasant Surprise of No False Flags

Experts often caution that whole-body scans can lead to numerous false positives, or "false flags," which are suspicious or indeterminate lesions that turn out benign. These false flags can cause unnecessary anxiety and lead to further invasive testing. With this in mind, I approached my first whole-body MRI scan with caution and nervousness, fully expecting to encounter a lot of suspicious and indeterminate findings in my body.

To my pleasant surprise, the results defied my expectations. While Prenuvo's whole-body MRI scan detected a few benign cysts at various sizes in my liver and kidneys, no suspicious or indeterminate lesions were found. This outcome challenges the common belief that false positives are an unavoidable aspect of preventive whole-body MRI scans. My scan's absence of false positives can be attributed to advancements in MRI technology and meticulously designed protocols. Modern MRI machines offer higher-resolution imaging and improved software algorithms, enabling precise differentiation between benign and potentially malignant lesions. These technological improvements reduce the likelihood of misinterpretation and false positives.

Moreover, using multiple scanning sequences during whole-body MRI scans is crucial in minimizing false positives. For example, T1-weighted sequences provide clear images of anatomical structures, while T2-weighted sequences are more sensitive to water content and can highlight abnormalities like cysts and tumors. Advanced imaging techniques, such as Diffusion-Weighted Imaging (DWI), have further enhanced the diagnostic accuracy of MRI scans. By combining these sequences, radiologists can cross-reference findings and make more accurate interpretations, reducing the chances of mistaking benign cysts or other non-threatening abnormalities for suspicious lesions.

Despite detecting multiple cysts, my experience of having no suspicious or indeterminate lesions illustrates the progress made in this field. This pleasant surprise reinforces the value of preventive whole-body imaging and its role in proactive early detection and preventive care. Of course, this is only my personal experience. The potential for false positives in preventive whole-body MRI scans remains a concern.

Comparative Experience with Ezra

Despite not detecting any suspicious or indeterminate lesions in my initial scan with Prenuvo, I opted to undergo a second whole-body MRI six months later at a different facility. This decision allowed me to compare the scan data and evaluate the technology's reliability.

For my second scan, I chose Ezra Scan's MRI service. Positioned as an accessible option in preventive screening, Ezra provides a unique yet equally impactful experience with their AI-assisted technology, which aims to make MRI scans faster and more affordable without compromising quality.

I selected its Full Body Plus option, which includes a whole-body MRI and a low-dose chest CT scan at a cost of $2,500. While MRI is increasingly used to detect pulmonary nodules, low-dose chest CT remains the gold standard for lung cancer screening. I wanted to compare the results of the whole-body MRI with those of the chest CT scan.

My interaction with Ezra was marked by professionalism and state-of-the-art imaging technology. I scheduled my whole-body MRI scan at one of Ezra's partner facilities, the RadNet Beverly Tower Wilshire Advanced Imaging Center in Los Angeles, CA. The scan was conducted using a GE Discovery 3T Tesla MRI Scanner on 05/26/2023.

A week later, on 06/01/2023, I received the Ezra Scan Report via email. The report was presented in a PDF file and also available online through my Ezra account. The PDF included a Table of Contents, Overall Impression, Detailed Findings of Body Sections, and Next Steps.

Overall Impression

In your Ezra Scan, which gives a view inside your body and looks for early disease and cancer, there were non-urgent findings that require follow-up. Please review the entire report and "Next Steps" for more details about all your findings. Connect with Ezra in 1 year to monitor your health.

The Overall Impression section of my report is shown here:

Techniques used to scan various body parts were provided in the detailed reports.

EXAM: MRI HEAD, NECK AND SPINE SCREENING WITHOUT CONTRAST (EZRA PROTOCOL)

HISTORY: Screening

COMPARISON: None available.

TECHNIQUE: Examination was performed on a GE Discovery 3T Tesla MRI scanner. Multiplanar MR imaging of the brain, neck, cervical spine, thoracic spine and lumbar spine was performed.

EXAM: MRI INFERIOR CHEST/ABDOMEN (PORTION OF WHOLE BODY SCAN) WITHOUT CONTRAST

HISTORY: Health screening exam

TECHNIQUE: The exam was performed on a GE Discovery 3T. Multiplanar MR imaging of the inferior chest and abdomen are performed including T1, T2, DWI, ADC, GRE sequences.

EXAM: MRI PROSTATE BI-PARAMETRIC

TECHNIQUE: Using a 3 Tesla MRI and a phased array coil, high resolution, small field-of-view imaging of the prostate was performed using the following sequences; axial T2-weighted, sagittal T2-weighted, oblique coronal T2-weighted, multiple b-value diffusion-weighted.

The section at the end of the report included the following statement: "Please note, the Ezra Service is for wellness purposes only. The Ezra Service is not diagnostic and does not replace currently accepted cancer screening standards (such as colonoscopy, mammography, etc.). Only organs and anatomy outlined in the report were reviewed as part of the Ezra Service. Please remember, it is the member's responsibility to arrange and act upon any of the included recommendations in this report."

I was pleased to find that Ezra's whole-body MRI scan detected the same cysts in my liver and kidneys, as well as other numerous degenerative changes in my shoulders, spine, and other parts. The CT and MRI scans yielded consistent results, reporting no pulmonary nodules.

The uniformity of the whole-body MRI findings from two different providers certainly enhances my confidence in this safe and sensitive imaging tool for preventive care.

Experiences of Whole-body MRI by Others

Preventive whole-body MRI has transformed early cancer detection, offering peace of mind and, at times, life-saving diagnoses. Here are personal stories from individuals who have experienced this procedure:

Maria's Story:

Maria Menounos, a renowned television presenter, shares her compelling journey with whole-body MRI screening, which has been pivotal in her health and wellness. In 2023, her life was altered by a startling discovery: a mass on her pancreas, identified through Prenuvo's whole-body MRI. Subsequent tests revealed Maria, at 44, had stage 2 pancreatic cancer, a disease notoriously elusive in its early stages. This diagnosis followed her recovery from a benign brain tumor in 2017, also discovered through proactive health measures.

Maria openly credits the whole-body MRI for catching the cancer early, before it advanced to a more severe stage. Typically, pancreatic cancer is only found once symptoms appear and the disease is more advanced; thus, the MRI's early intervention significantly enhanced her treatment options and prognosis. Her story highlights the importance of proactive health screenings, particularly with advanced imaging technologies like whole-body MRI, which can uncover abnormalities before symptoms arise. Maria Menounos's narrative has inspired many to consider the life-saving potential of such screenings, especially for cancers that are hard to detect early. By sharing her experience, she has raised awareness about the critical role of early detection and the value of whole-body MRI in preventive healthcare, showcasing how these technologies can detect serious illnesses early when they are most treatable.

Michael's Story:

Michael, a 55-year-old executive, opted for a whole-body MRI as part of his annual health check-up. Despite being asymptomatic and generally healthy, he wanted to address potential health issues proactively. The MRI uncovered a small tumor in his pancreas that had not yet caused symptoms. Early detection enabled Michael to undergo timely surgery, removing the cancer before it spread. His experience underscores the crucial role of early detection and how preventive measures like whole-body MRI can distinguish between a routine procedure and a severe health crisis.

Laura's Journey:

Laura, a 48-year-old teacher with a family history of cancer but no personal symptoms, was encouraged by her family and doctor to have a whole-body MRI as a precautionary step. The scan revealed a mass in her bile duct, an area challenging to monitor with routine checks. Further tests confirmed it was early-stage bile duct cancer, a condition often undetected until advanced. Laura's early diagnosis allowed for successful treatment, and she now advocates for whole-body MRI as a preventive tool, especially for those with a family history of cancer.

Tom's Experience:

Tom, a 60-year-old fitness enthusiast, firmly believed in regular health screenings. Embracing a proactive approach to well-being, he chose to undergo a whole-body MRI. This decision proved crucial as it revealed a small, early-stage tumor in his small intestine—a location where cancer is often only detected at advanced stages. Thanks to this early discovery, Tom received timely treatment, significantly improving his prognosis. Tom's experience highlights the invaluable role of whole-body MRI in identifying cancers that are typically elusive in their early stages.

Susan's Revelation:

Susan, a 52-year-old marketing consultant, was prompted by a colleague's battle with cancer to take her health more seriously. Though asymptomatic, she opted for a whole-body MRI. The scan detected an early-stage ovarian cancer, a type notoriously difficult to catch early. Susan commenced treatment immediately and attributed the whole-body MRI with potentially saving her life by identifying the tumor before it could advance.

These stories underscore the transformative potential of preventive whole-body MRI. Despite differing motivations and outcomes, the common theme is the critical importance of early detection. For many, whole-body MRI presents an opportunity for early intervention, often before symptoms emerge, leading to improved treatment outcomes and saving lives.

Navigating Whole-body MRI: A Journey of Health Consciousness

Undergoing a preventive whole-body MRI scan was a profoundly proactive decision for my well-being, shedding light on the intricate relationship between technology and preventive care. This journey introduced me to two exceptional providers, each offering unique experiences.

My initial encounter was with a leading preventive MRI provider renowned for its combination of advanced technology and compassionate healthcare. Their imaging quality and thorough follow-up were outstanding, but what truly defined my experience was the attention to customer service and the serene environment of the imaging center.

Ezra, the second provider, offered a fresh take on preventive care. Their innovative use of technology to enhance patient service was noteworthy. While maintaining high standards in imaging and follow-up, their distinct approach to customer care and the welcoming atmosphere of their center provided a different yet equally valuable experience.

These scans not only gave me a snapshot of my current health but also established a baseline for future monitoring, empowering me to make informed decisions about preventive care. My experiences highlight the potential of whole-body MRI exams to ease anxiety, detect issues early, and guide proactive health choices.

Choosing whole-body MRI for early cancer detection was a profoundly personal journey, balancing emotional and rational factors. It was as much about self-awareness as it was about the marvels of medical technology. Awaiting results was an emotionally charged experience, but the findings brought a sense of calm, reinforcing my control over my future health, regardless of the outcome.

Reflecting on this journey, the decision to undergo a proactive whole-body MRI symbolizes a broader narrative—facing the unknown, taking control of our well-being, and embracing preventive care for early detection of cancer and other medical conditions.

Future Direction: Maximizing Early Detection, Minimizing Potential Harm

Preventive systemic cancer screening with whole-body MRI scans is still in its infancy, with considerable room for enhancement. Here are several areas for improvement:

Navigating Indeterminate and Suspicious Findings: Systemic Screening and Local Monitoring. A pivotal aspect of systemic early cancer detection is managing test results, particularly indeterminate and suspicious findings. Indeterminate findings, which are neither clearly benign nor malignant, often necessitate further investigation, leading to additional imaging or biopsies. This process can be stressful and costly for patients. The ambiguity of such results can also lead to overdiagnosis and overtreatment, particularly in cancers like thyroid and prostate, where aggressive treatments may not improve survival and can negatively impact quality of life. Localized monitoring with CT or MRI should be used to examine specific areas of concern identified by systemic screening. For instance, if a whole-body MRI detects a suspicious lesion in the liver, a follow-up local MRI or CT can offer detailed insights into the lesion's characteristics, aiding in distinguishing benign from malignant features. Standardized protocols can help determine which findings are likely clinically significant and when to follow up on them, reducing overdiagnosis and overtreatment—common pitfalls in early detection.

Standardizing Protocols: A primary concern in early cancer detection tests is the specificity, sensitivity, and reproducibility of tests. Optimizing and standardizing protocols are crucial to minimizing false positives and negatives, which can lead to unnecessary anxiety, follow-up tests, or missed diagnoses. Such standardization ensures consistent, reliable test results that are comparable over time and across different clinical environments.

Managing Fear and Mental Stress: The emotional impact of undergoing screening tests is significant. Pre- and post-scan counseling becomes a vital component of the diagnostic process, preparing patients for the possibility of indeterminate findings, which are not uncommon in extensive scans. Counseling helps manage the fear and mental stress associated with such results.

Undergoing an MRI scan can be daunting, leading to "scanxiety," a term describing the anxiety and fear associated with the procedure, its results, or the confined space of the MRI machine. This psychological impact, including stress and anxiety related to test findings, is a significant pitfall of preventive whole-body MRI. To mitigate this, comprehensive education and counseling should be integral to the screening process. Individuals should be well-informed about potential scan outcomes, including incidental findings and their implications. Pre-scan consultations can help manage expectations and reduce anxiety, while post-scan follow-ups with healthcare professionals can provide clarity and support in interpreting results. It is essential to assess an individual's capacity to handle potentially ambiguous or concerning findings before they undergo such testing.

Individuals unable to calmly and methodically manage the uncertainty of indeterminate and suspicious findings are not suitable for these systemic screening tests. Acting hastily on follow-up examinations can do more harm than good. A significant portion of lesions detected by whole-body MRI are benign or indolent, and the psychological impact could be profound and counterproductive to overall wellbeing.

Enhance Imaging Quality Further. Improving imaging quality is pivotal for maximizing the utility of whole-body MRI in preventive care. Advances in MRI technology, such as higher field strengths and superior coil designs, can yield clearer, more detailed images. This is especially important for detecting early signs of disease, such as small tumors or subtle changes in soft tissue structure, which may be missed with less advanced imaging systems.

Conduct Randomized Controlled Trials: Randomized controlled trials are needed to demonstrate the positive predictive value (PPV) of whole-body MRI scans and the reduction of cancer-related deaths. These trials should compare health outcomes between populations receiving regular MRI scans and those who do not, providing robust data on the benefits of MRI in preventive care. Such evidence is crucial for convincing healthcare providers and government agencies to support widespread preventive MRI screening programs.

Cost Reduction to Increase Accessibility and Equality: A significant barrier to the widespread adoption of proactive whole-body MRIs is their high cost. Currently, these scans are not covered by insurance but can be paid for using Health Savings Accounts (HSA) and Flexible Spending Accounts (FSA). Companies like Prenuvo and Ezra are working to make these services more accessible and affordable. Prenuvo aims to significantly reduce the cost of their scans, democratizing access to advanced diagnostic imaging and improving public health. SimonONE currently offers a basic MRI scan option covering major organs at a price of approximately $650 to $950.

More importantly, rapid advances in AI and technology have the potential to reduce MRI scan costs significantly. For example, AI-enhanced low-cost MRI scanners and scanning protocols have shown great promise in cost reduction. The Ezra Full Body MRI, which previously took one hour and cost $1,950, is now available as a 30-minute AI-assisted full-body MRI scan for $1,350. Ezra hopes to offer a $500 15-minute full-body scan in the near future. These developments highlight significant strides in making preventive care more accessible and cost-effective, though it is crucial to ensure that cost reductions do not compromise image quality.

Choose Quality Service Providers: The efficacy of whole-body MRI scans and other diagnostic tests heavily depends on the quality of the service provider. Opting for facilities and professionals that uphold high standards, possess the necessary certifications, and utilize up-to-date technology is crucial. A top-tier service provider not only ensures precise findings but also enhances the overall experience through skilled staff, effective communication, and efficient processes. I have been impressed with the whole-body MRI services offered by Prenuvo and Ezra.

Personally, I believe the potential pitfalls of these systemic early detection tests can be effectively mitigated by proceeding methodically when encountering suspicious or indeterminate findings. Even opting for a follow-up examination, such as a local CT or PET/CT, to determine whether a suspicious lesion is inactive or benign is worthwhile. Such follow-up examinations are preferable to the symptom-triggered diagnosis of advanced, incurable cancer.

In summary, whole-body MRI scans are increasingly recognized as powerful tools for early disease detection and intervention as preventive care gains traction. Introducing and adopting new cancer screening tests is a lengthy and complex process. This journey can be particularly challenging during transitional periods when scientific research and policy have not aligned with technological advancements. Andrew Lacy, founder and CEO of Prenuvo, points out the protracted journey of mammograms before they gained acceptance. Although mammograms became popular in the 1960s, they were not endorsed by the American Cancer Society until 1976 and were not covered by insurance until the 1990s. Similarly, it may take time for whole-body MRI to achieve widespread acceptance and utilization in preventive care.

With its proven sensitivity and rapid improvement through AI integration, whole-body MRI has the potential to become the most effective tool for identifying minuscule precancerous and cancerous lesions at early curable stages, as well as other abnormalities throughout the entire body. This positions it as an indispensable tool for early disease detection, pivotal for personalized preventive care for cancer and other diseases.

Without any financial ties to MRI service providers or imaging centers, I am genuinely captivated by the unparalleled potential of whole-body MRI in early disease detection. It has the power to transform the current ineffective, reactive 'sick care' system into a proactive healthcare model. The key challenges affecting the timely adoption of preventive whole-body MRI are further explored in the following chapters.

Transforming Systemic Early Detection with AI

CHAPTER EIGHT

"AI will be part of every industry, enhancing our abilities in ways we can't even imagine yet."
Jeff Bezos

"AI and generative AI may be the most important technology of any lifetime."
Marc Benioff

How can we improve the accuracy, sensitivity, and effectiveness of these sophisticated systemic early detection tests?

A profound transformation has emerged in the vast expanse of scientific exploration, driven by the enigmatic world of artificial intelligence (AI).

AI has journeyed from a science fiction concept to a pivotal force spurring innovation and transformation across every sector of our society. The idea of intelligent artificial beings dates back to ancient myths and legends, but the formal study of AI began in the mid-20th century. British mathematician and logician Alan Turing laid the groundwork with his seminal 1950 paper "Computing Machinery and Intelligence," where he asked, "Can machines think?"

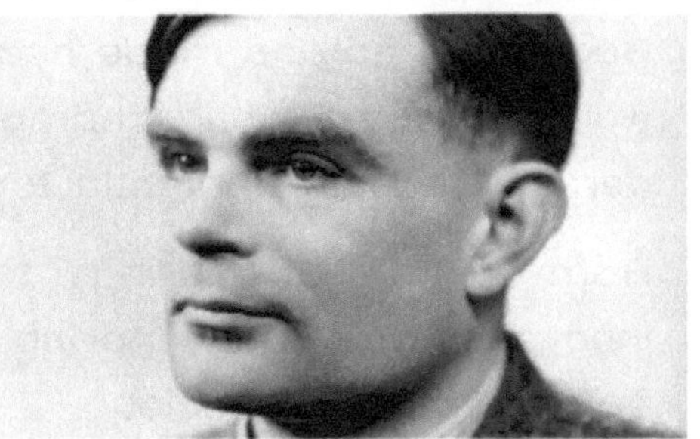

A photograph of Alan Turing, 1951. Source: Royal British Legion

He introduced the Turing Test, a measure of a machine's ability to exhibit human-like intelligence.

The term "artificial intelligence" was coined in 1956 by American computer scientist John McCarthy during the

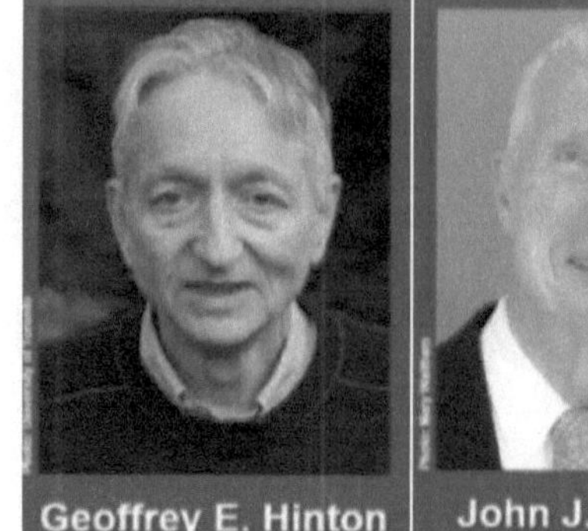
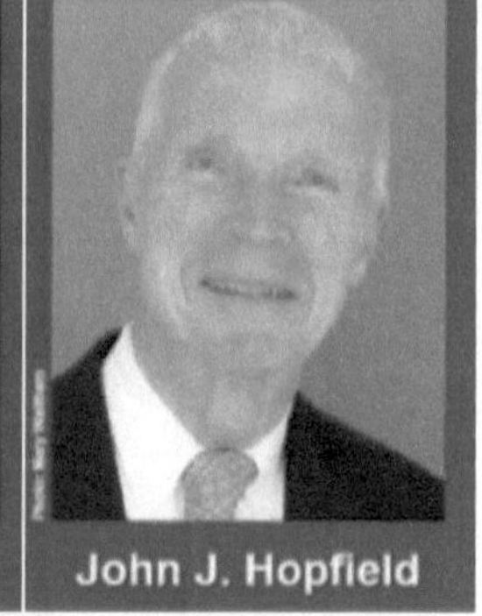

Geoffrey E. Hinton | John J. Hopfield

Nobel Prize Winners in Physics in 2024

Dartmouth Conference, an event often considered the birth of AI as a distinct field of study.

The 1950s and 1960s saw the development of early AI programs. However, when early promises of the field turned out to be over-ambitious, initial excitement gave way to what has been described as an "AI Winter," a period defined by diminished interest and funding. The 1990s and 2000s saw the dawn of machine learning, a subfield interested in making computers learn from data using algorithms. This change was enabled in part by the explosion of worldwide computational power and big data. IBM's Deep Blue was the most successful AI of that period, capable of defeating a world chess champion, Garry Kasparov, in 1997.

The late 2000s and 2010s saw the rise of deep learning, a subset of machine learning involving neural networks with many layers, which were pioneered by John Hopfield and Geoffrey Hinton, winners of the 2024 Nobel Prize in Physics. AI has become ubiquitous in the last decade, driving advancements in many fields, such as healthcare, transportation, and entertainment. Google's DeepMind made headlines with its AlphaGo program, which defeated world champion Go player Lee Sedol in 2016, demonstrating AI's potential to tackle complex problems.

From theoretical musings to practical applications, the AI innovation train is now moving at a breathtaking pace, impacting every corner of our society.

Entering a New AI Era

2023 marked a pivotal moment when AI's transformative capabilities profoundly reshaped industries and societies. At the forefront of this revolution stood generative AI, an innovative subset renowned for its remarkable ability to mimic human creativity and intelligence, producing content that spans text, imagery, and beyond.

The rise of machine learning models and exponential increases in computational power and access to massive amounts of data have enabled AI systems to digest massive information, recognize patterns, and minimize human intervention when making decisions. Consequently, AI has graduated from a niche technology to an enabler of strategic growth across industries worldwide.

The AI revolution is mainly due to realizing some significant steps in natural language understanding (NLU) and generative AI. These technologies have converged on what a machine can do and given an interface that people can interact with. NLU systems can understand the languages that humans use. In unison, generative AI has emerged as transformative technology able to create content—from text to images— that looks nearly indistinguishable from human-created work. These developments reveal the breadth of AI and how it can reshape industries by facilitating creativity, efficiency, and decision-making.

The Rise of Generative AI

Generative AI represents a significant step forward in how machines learn and can generate utterly original content across various dimensions (words, images, sounds) and purposefully mimic human-like creative behaviors. In contrast to traditional AI, which is more about analyses and data interpretation, generative AI allows someone to create based on learned patterns/structures. Here, I briefly summarize the features of generative AI.

Unmatched Creativity. Generative AI leads us into an era where the limits of space and time for creativity are stretched to unknown maximums. It enlivens countless types of human expression, from the visual grandeur in art to music so poignant it touches our spirits most divinely and even writing that transcends the possibilities we could ever dream up. With this kind of genius, we are opened to extraordinary possibilities. AI-driven creativity can transform the work of architecture, fashion, medicine, and product development, liberate conventional design thinking, and spur innovation.

Unparalleled Efficiency and Productivity. AI automates manual and time-consuming work in ways that are implausible with human beings, thus leading to an unprecedentedly increased level of productivity across numerous sectors. AI can do everything from creating complex code to producing appealing marketing narratives. Intelligent AI, the so-called 'biorobots,' will reduce operational costs and improve resource allocation, ushering in a new era of economy and welfare on a global scale.

Personalization and Customization. AI can tailor experiences and products that analyze personal tastes & behavior. Specific solutions at the dawn of marketing, care, and education improvement user participation rise to chase unprecedented outcomes. Furthermore, the fact that AI learns and improves with each new exposure translates into ever more nuanced responses — an excellent rendition of adaptive intelligence.

Unmatched Problem-Solving with Complex Data Analysis and Prediction. Generative AI is highly efficient in sifting through that dataset to find the most intricate patterns even the smartest human mind may miss.

In summary, generative AI is a true breakthrough in artificial intelligence, with immense potential to disrupt several domains by being able to generate entirely novel and intricate content.

Generative AI will become more and more of the driving force behind what creativity in innovation and problem-solving looks like for us, leading humanity toward a better future.

Technological Foundations of AI Breakthroughs

The Essential Role of GPUs in AI

Over the past decades, it has been an exciting journey for us as elements like graphic processing units (GPUs) surfaced with evolving capabilities of these architectures to boost this technology significantly. Initially developed to render video game graphics, GPUs have very purposefully moved beyond this initial application as a critical driver of the growth in AI and machine learning (ML), powered by efficient, parallel processing capabilities. This architectural design enables thousands of small cores to handle many tasks simultaneously. Because of this property, GPUs excel at large-scale matrix and vector operations, on which many AI apps rest.

NVIDIA, founded and headed by CEO Jensen Huang, has been a central underpinning of this transformational saga with the development of the CUDA (Compute Unified

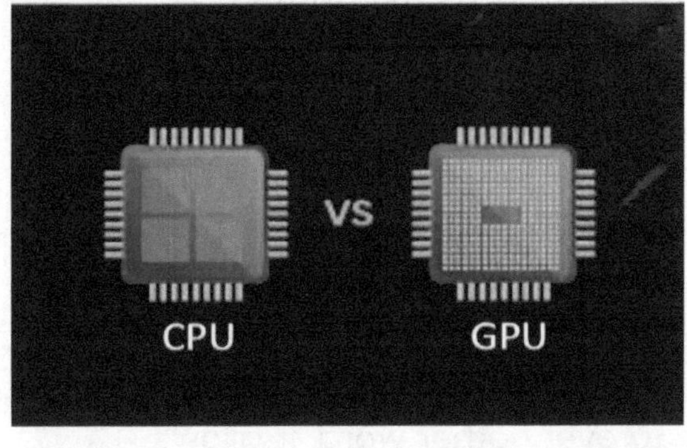

Device Architecture) platform seeing use for GPGPU (General Purpose computing on GPUs) capabilities. This innovation was instrumental for AI and deep learning workloads, resulting in increased productivity as these types of machine learning models need enormous datasets to be processed quicker than the time it would require before training. Thus, GPUs have become essential to every AI infrastructure deployed anywhere.

Transformer Models in AI

The relentless advancement of computational power, driven by the progression of GPUs, has spurred the development of increasingly sophisticated and efficient machine learning algorithms. Deep learning, characterized by neural networks with multiple layers, has particularly thrived thanks to these advancements.

The transformer architecture, introduced by Vaswani et al. from Google in their 2017 groundbreaking paper "Attention is All You Need," has revolutionized the AI field, particularly in natural language processing (NLP) and generative AI. This innovative architecture addressed many challenges of previous models, such as recurrent neural networks (RNNs) and convolutional neural networks (CNNs), delivering unparalleled performance and versatility.

Built on self-attention mechanisms, the transformer architecture processes input data more efficiently and effectively than traditional models. The self-attention mechanism calculates attention scores for each word in a sequence relative to every other word. It allows the model to weigh the importance of different words

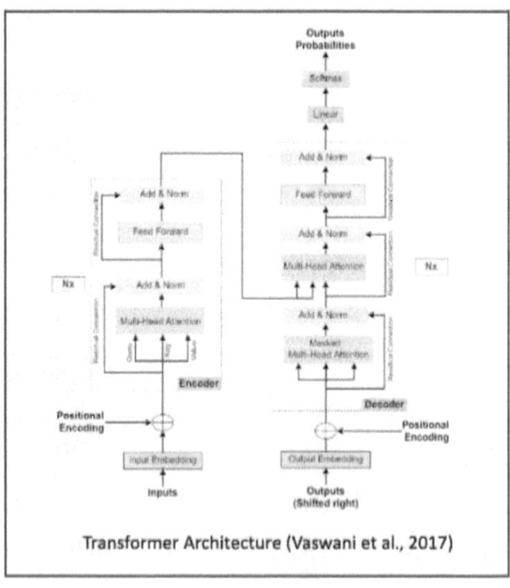

Transformer Architecture (Vaswani et al., 2017)

based on their contextual relationships. This capability captures long-range dependencies and enhances understanding, setting a new standard for AI performance. Following each attention layer, a feed-forward neural network awaits, composed of linear transformations and nonlinear activations. These networks apply complex transformations to the data, enabling the model to learn and discern intricate patterns that would otherwise remain elusive. They act as the alchemists of information, transmuting raw data into refined understanding.

The transformer architecture has ushered in a renaissance of generative AI, offering several key advantages that have reshaped the landscape:

- **Elevated Performance**: Transformer models can process entire sequences simultaneously. This makes them more computationally efficient and better suited for parallel processing. The self-attention mechanism allows transformer models to capture long-range dependencies more effectively, improving accuracy in language modeling and generation tasks.

- **Scalability**: Transformer models can be scaled up to create colossal models, which have achieved unprecedented heights across various natural language processing benchmarks. These pre-trained transformer models can be fine-tuned for specific tasks, leveraging the knowledge gained from training on immense datasets.

- **Versatility**: Transformer models are true polymaths, adaptable to various generative tasks, from text generation and translation to summarization and image and music generation. The architecture has been successfully applied to domains far beyond text, such as vision (Vision Transformers) and protein folding (AlphaFold), demonstrating its versatility and boundless potential.

So, to sum it up, the transformer architecture introduced by Vaswani et al. has changed the realm of generative AI. Its innovative self-attention mechanism and scalable architecture have catalyzed significant performance, efficiency, and versatility advancements. Transformer models have revolutionized applications in text generation, machine translation, text summarization, and beyond, setting new benchmarks in AI. As research continues to evolve, transformer models stand poised to drive further innovations, unlocking new possibilities in AI and transforming diverse fields with their generative capabilities. The era of transformers is indeed upon us.

Large Language Models: Pioneers of the New Age

Large language models (LLM) are some of the most groundbreaking advancements in AI capabilities. As evidenced by ChatGPT, these models sit atop incredible language generals for their understanding of and ability to produce human-like text that is more fluent and coherent than ever before. The Generative Pre-Trained Transformer (GPT) arranges a new high-water mark for what AI can understand in human language.

The evolution of OpenAI's chat models has been remarkable, rapidly progressing from ChatGPT-2 to ChatGPT-4. Introduced in 2019, ChatGPT-2 was already noteworthy for its capability to generate coherent and contextually relevant text from given prompts, utilizing a state-of-the-art language model with 1.5 billion parameters. Despite its strengths, it had limited response accuracy, contextual understanding, and nuanced content generation—areas significantly improved in subsequent versions.

That made way for ChatGPT-4, released in 2023. This iteration passed the 100 trillion parameter mark. It led to a noticeable improvement in enabling models to understand and generate human-like text across many more topics in additional languages. It also included enhancements like better reasoning capabilities, style adaptation, and the ability to manage complicated questions. In addition, ChatGPT-4 came with better safeguards and bolstered training techniques to help foster more precise answers that are contextually sound as well as safer interactions. These improvements further established its use cases, from educational tools to customer service solutions.

Moreover, GPT-4o, a multilingual and multimodal generative pre-trained transformer designed by OpenAI, was released on May 13, 2024. GPT-4o set new benchmarks in voice, multilingual, and vision tasks, achieving state-of-the-art audio speech recognition and translation results. By combining big data insights with improvements in LLM, we are on the edge of these new AI applications. They are expected to revolutionize every aspect of our lives. They promise to entirely reinvent not just individual industries but also society as a whole.

AI in Transforming Healthcare: An Overview

AI is set to revolutionize healthcare, ushering in a new era of personalized, efficient, and data-driven medical care. Integrating AI into various healthcare sectors promises significant improvements in patient outcomes, operational efficiency, and global health challenges.

"We've witnessed the dawn of a true transformation in the healthcare industry with the power of AI," wrote Scott Miller, Chief Marketing Officer of Imaging at GE Healthcare.

One of AI's most profound impacts in healthcare is enhancing clinical decision-making and enabling personalized medicine. AI algorithms can analyze vast amounts of patient data, including medical records, genomic information, and real-time monitoring data, providing clinicians with valuable insights and recommendations. This leads to more accurate diagnoses, tailored treatment plans, and improved patient outcomes.

For example, AI-powered diagnostic tools can more accurately analyze medical images, such as X-rays and MRI scans, than human experts. These tools detect subtle patterns and anomalies that may be missed by the naked eye, assisting radiologists and pathologists in making precise diagnoses, reducing the risk of misdiagnosis, and enabling earlier interventions.

AI is revolutionizing healthcare by predicting disease progression and treatment outcomes, enabling personalized therapies tailored to individual genetics, lifestyles, and medical histories. This innovative approach enhances treatment effectiveness, minimizes side effects, and improves overall patient care. Additionally, AI streamlines administrative tasks such as scheduling, record management, and insurance processing, allowing healthcare professionals to focus more on patient interactions.

Beyond enhancing patient care, AI optimizes hospital operations by improving patient flow and resource allocation. Predictive analytics can forecast patient demand and identify potential bottlenecks, leading to more efficient resource utilization and shorter wait times. In public health, AI analyzes extensive data sets to uncover patterns, anticipate outbreaks, and guide targeted interventions, empowering authorities to respond more effectively to health threats.

Integrating AI with wearable devices and telemedicine platforms transforms patient monitoring and care delivery. AI-powered wearables track vital signs and health indicators, providing real-time insights and early warnings for proactive interventions. Virtual care assistants offer personalized health advice, medication reminders, and triage services, alleviating some burdens on healthcare providers.

However, addressing ethical challenges is crucial to harnessing AI's full potential in healthcare. This necessitates collaboration among providers, policymakers, and technology developers to ensure AI's responsible and equitable deployment, ultimately leading to a more accessible, efficient, and personalized healthcare system.

AI in Medical Diagnostics

AI in medical diagnostics presents a multitude of advantages, such as accelerated diagnosis and intervention, enhanced precision medicine, and a reduced workload for healthcare practitioners. AI technology empowers medical professionals to identify conditions, facilitating early interventions swiftly. It also plays a vital role in monitoring patients by detecting even the slightest changes in extensive data sets. Integrating AI into medical imaging significantly improves the accuracy of precision medicine, enabling tailored therapies based on specific disease types. Furthermore, AI-driven medical imaging analysis shortens diagnosis times, alleviating workplace burnout among healthcare providers and addressing the global shortage of medical specialists.

AI Image Recognition: Surpassing Human Capabilities

AI image recognition has emerged as a transformative technology with profound implications in the digital age. From healthcare to security, AI's rapid analysis of vast amounts of visual data surpasses human capabilities, opening new frontiers in efficiency, accuracy, and innovation.

AI image recognition involves using algorithms and neural networks trained to interpret and understand the content of digital images. This technology can identify objects, faces, scenes, and activities in pictures and videos, much like the human eye, but at a scale and speed unimaginable for humans. The process starts with data input, where numerous images are fed into the AI system to "train" it. Over time, these systems learn to recognize patterns and features more accurately.

The most significant advantage of AI image recognition is its speed and efficiency in processing large datasets. While humans can interpret intricate images, they cannot match AI systems' high-speed processing. For instance, in medical diagnostics, AI can scan thousands of medical images when it takes a radiologist to evaluate one. This swift processing saves time and identifies patterns the human eye might miss. AI also offers a consistency that human analysis cannot always match. While humans might get tired or be influenced by subjective biases, an AI system remains objective and consistent, provided it has been trained on a diverse and representative dataset.

The applications of AI image recognition are diverse and transformative. In healthcare, AI aids in early disease detection, such as cancer, by analyzing MRIs and identifying subtle signs of disease more accurately and efficiently than human practitioners.

The NVIDIA Clara Platform: AI Integration into Medical Imaging and Healthcare

The NVIDIA Clara Platform seamlessly integrates artificial intelligence and high-performance computing to revolutionize healthcare and life sciences. Its mission is to enhance medical imaging, genomics, and smart medical instruments, paving the way for unprecedented advancements in these sectors.

Clara significantly improves medical imaging techniques such as MRI, CT scans, and X-rays. With its AI-driven capabilities, Clara rapidly and accurately analyzes vast datasets, enabling the detection and diagnosis of conditions that may elude the human eye. This efficiency reduces interpretation time, ensuring timely and effective patient care.

Clara also plays a vital role in the development of intelligent medical instruments. These sophisticated devices utilize AI algorithms and sensors for real-time monitoring and analysis of patient data. From intelligent ultrasound machines to AI-enhanced endoscopy tools, Clara empowers these instruments to deliver precise and reliable patient care.

With its modular and scalable architecture, including the Clara Deploy component, Clara facilitates the seamless integration of AI applications into clinical workflows. This fosters a collaborative ecosystem for innovation, allowing healthcare providers to adopt AI solutions that directly enhance patient care.

By combining the NVIDIA Clara Platform with the DGX Cloud, healthcare organizations gain robust tools for developing and deploying medical imaging AI applications. Clara provides the necessary frameworks, while the DGX Cloud delivers scalability and computational power. This collaboration enhances diagnostic processes, leveraging AI and human expertise to refine medical imaging analysis, ultimately improving patient outcomes and advancing medical research.

AI in Transforming MRI

In the ever-evolving landscape of medical science, a revolution is underway, where AI is redefining the way, we perceive and analyze medical images. These sophisticated algorithms, born from the synergy of machine learning and deep learning, possess a remarkable ability to decode intricate patterns and features hidden within extensive datasets.

One area where AI's potential is particularly evident is in the analysis of MRI scans. Like a meticulous apprentice, AI models are rigorously trained on vast collections of meticulously labeled images, sharpening their ability to recognize subtle indicators of various conditions. Once fully trained, these intelligent systems assist radiologists by scrutinizing images and highlighting areas of concern with unwavering precision.

The development and training of AI systems on extensive datasets equip them with the capability to identify subtle patterns indicative of malignancy. This approach significantly enhances the reliability of whole-body MRI scans in cancer detection, leading to improved patient outcomes. Furthermore, AI algorithms can measure nodule size, boundary features, density, and heterogeneity, aiding in differentiating between benign and malignant lesions. This data-driven approach reduces reliance on subjective interpretation and boosts diagnostic accuracy.

AI's guidance makes the diagnostic process swifter and more precise than ever. These intelligent algorithms can provide invaluable diagnostic suggestions and quantify the likelihood of malignancy, empowering healthcare professionals to make informed decisions and offer optimal patient care in various ways.

AI in Distinguishing Benign and Malignant Lesions

In medical diagnostics, one challenge stands out: distinguishing between benign and malignant lesions. This crucial task is vital for determining the appropriate follow-up tests and treatment course.

Benign lesions are non-cancerous and generally pose no apparent threat to one's wellbeing. Malignant lesions, however, signal a graver danger—cancer, a formidable adversary that can metastasize and spread throughout the body. Accurate differentiation between these two entities is essential, as it informs patient care strategies and maximizes the chances of a favorable outcome.

MRI is a powerful imaging modality that provides detailed images of soft tissues, making it invaluable in diagnosing various conditions, including tumors. MRI utilizes magnetic fields and radio waves to generate images, offering superior contrast resolution compared to other imaging techniques. Despite its advantages, interpreting MRI scans can be complex and time-consuming, often requiring highly trained radiologists. Moreover, MRI findings can sometimes be inconclusive, necessitating additional tests or biopsies, which can be invasive and costly.

AI algorithms can be trained to distinguish between benign and malignant lesions by analyzing various features in MRI scans. These features include lesion shape, size, margin characteristics, internal architecture, and signal intensity on different MRI sequences. For example, malignant lesions often exhibit irregular shapes, spiculated margins, and heterogeneous internal structures, whereas benign lesions tend to be more regular and homogeneous.

Deep learning models, particularly convolutional neural networks (CNNs), have demonstrated high accuracy in image classification tasks, including distinguishing between benign and malignant lesions. CNNs can automatically learn relevant features from raw image data without requiring manual feature extraction, making them exceptionally well-suited for medical imaging applications.

AI in Reducing Indeterminate Findings

In medical imaging, indeterminate findings on MRI scans have long been a cause of frustration and uncertainty, often resulting in additional diagnostic procedures and prolonged anxiety for patients. However, AI has emerged as a beacon of hope, offering numerous strategies to mitigate these indeterminate findings and provide more accurate and confident interpretations. The AI Advantage includes:

- **Enhanced Image Analysis:** AI can scrutinize subtle features in MRI scans that might escape even the most experienced human radiologists. AI comprehensively assesses lesions by integrating data from multiple MRI sequences and using advanced algorithms, reducing the likelihood of indeterminate findings.

- **Predictive Modeling:** By analyzing extensive datasets of MRI scans and associated clinical outcomes, AI can develop predictive models that quantify the probability of malignancy for a given lesion. This information enables radiologists to make more informed decisions, minimizing the need for follow-up tests and reducing patient burden.

- **Radiomics and Texture Analysis:** AI can extract quantitative features from medical images that reflect underlying pathophysiology—a field known as radiomics. Analyzing these features, AI can distinguish between benign and malignant lesions with unparalleled precision. Texture analysis, a subset of radiomics, examines the intricate patterns within lesions, offering additional insights that can resolve indeterminate findings.

- **Continuous Learning and Improvement:** AI systems continuously learn and improve by processing more data, unlike their human counterparts. This ability allows AI to adapt to new challenges and refine its diagnostic accuracy, reducing the incidence of indeterminate findings and enabling healthcare professionals to provide the best possible care.

- **Integration with Clinical Data:** AI systems can seamlessly integrate MRI findings with other clinical data, including patient history, laboratory results, and genetic information. This holistic approach provides a more complete picture of the patient's condition, enhancing diagnostic accuracy and reducing indeterminate findings.

The potential of AI in MRI diagnostics has already been demonstrated in several real-world applications and case studies, showcasing the transformative power of these technologies.

One such study, conducted by researchers at the University of California, highlighted the remarkable accuracy of an AI algorithm in classifying liver lesions on MRI scans. By analyzing the lesions' shape, texture, and enhancement patterns across different MRI sequences, the AI system significantly reduced the number of indeterminate cases, offering valuable clarity and direction for patient care.

Another notable success is in the detection and characterization of brain tumors. AI models have been developed to differentiate between primary brain tumors, metastatic lesions, and benign conditions such as meningiomas. These models have shown high accuracy in distinguishing these entities, providing invaluable support to radiologists, and reducing the need for invasive procedures like biopsies, alleviating the burden on patients and their families.

As the integration of AI in medical diagnostics continues to unfold, these technological advancements stand poised to revolutionize the field, ushering in a new era of precision, clarity, and compassionate care for all.

AI in Reducing Motion Artifacts in MRI

AI is crucial in minimizing motion artifacts in MRI scans, resulting in faster, higher-quality imaging. Advanced deep learning models, particularly convolutional neural networks, excel at detecting and assessing motion artifacts in real-time. This capability serves as a safeguard for AI-driven reconstructions, allowing for timely re-acquisition of images when necessary. Moreover, techniques such as conditional generative adversarial networks (CGANs) have proven effective in correcting these artifacts and reconstructing high-quality images from undersampled data. Research indicates that CGAN models enhance image quality and resilience against motion-related issues. Notably, researchers at MIT have developed a pioneering deep learning model that integrates physics-based modeling with neural networks to generate motion-free MRI images, ensuring data consistency and eliminating the risk of fabricated features. AI's proficiency in detecting, quantifying, and rectifying motion artifacts reduces scan times and costs while significantly improving diagnostic accuracy, particularly for patients who find it challenging to remain still.

AI in Enhancing the Accuracy of MRI Diagnostics

The accuracy of medical diagnostics is crucial, with a significant impact on patient outcomes. AI technologies, particularly those employing federated learning algorithms, have shown remarkable promise in enhancing the diagnostic accuracy of MRI scans. By training on a diverse dataset collected from multiple institutions, these AI models can learn various patterns and anomalies associated with different diseases.

The workload on radiologists has been steadily increasing due to the growing demand for imaging services and a global shortage of qualified professionals. With their autonomous learning capabilities, AI technologies present a viable solution to alleviate this burden. By automating the analysis and interpretation of MRI scans, AI can significantly reduce the time and effort required by radiologists to review each image manually.

Moreover, the use of AI in medical imaging extends beyond mere analysis; it can also assist in the tedious task of annotating images, identifying relevant features, and even prioritizing cases based on urgency. This reduced workload allows radiologists to focus more on complex cases requiring expert judgment, thus enhancing the overall quality of patient care. Additionally, alleviating manual tasks reduces burnout among radiologists, addressing a critical issue in the healthcare workforce.

Recent advancements in AI have heralded a new era of diagnostic precision in medical imaging. One notable development is the integration of AI technology to enhance MRI analysis.

A prime example is the creation of a federated AI algorithm for brain MRI scans. Developed collaboratively by researchers from Helmholtz Munich, Technical University of Munich, and University Hospital Bonn, this "self-learning" algorithm signifies a significant leap in medical imaging. It is trained across various medical institutions without requiring extensive radiologist annotations, thus preserving data privacy and accelerating learning. The algorithm's capacity to autonomously learn from over 1,500 MR scans of healthy individuals and accurately identify diseases such as multiple sclerosis and various brain tumors marks a pivotal advancement in AI-driven diagnostics.

Recently, the FDA cleared a groundbreaking AI software called Sonic DL from GE Healthcare, which can reduce cardiac MRI scan times by up to 83%. Sonic DL employs deep learning technology to facilitate cardiac MRI scans 12 times faster than conventional systems, enabling high-quality imaging within a single heartbeat—an unprecedented feat. By leveraging AI reconstruction from limited data, Sonic DL drastically improves radiology workflow efficiency, alleviates backlogs, and potentially broadens patient eligibility for cardiac MRI. The accelerated scanning process enhances accessibility and comfort for patients with breath-holding, advanced heart failure, or arrhythmias. AI-reconstructed images generated by Sonic DL are diagnostically equivalent to those from conventional lengthy MRI scans. This FDA clearance is viewed as a game-changer in cardiac imaging, addressing unique patient challenges while improving workflow and expanding access to this vital diagnostic tool.

Moreover, AI can significantly reduce MRI scanning times while maintaining diagnostic image quality. The core principle involves using AI to intelligently synthesize missing data from accelerated partial MRI acquisitions, drastically cutting scan times without compromising image quality. This AI-accelerated MRI approach can potentially increase patient comfort, improve accessibility, reduce costs, and enhance efficiency in MRI imaging.

Challenges of AI in MRI Diagnostics

Integrating AI into existing medical systems presents significant logistical and technical hurdles. Many healthcare institutions rely on legacy systems incompatible with emerging AI technologies. Upgrading these systems demands substantial investment, expertise, and time. Furthermore, interoperability remains critical, as various institutions employ diverse software and hardware configurations. Ensuring that AI algorithms function seamlessly across these different systems necessitates standardization in both technical compatibility and clinical workflows.

The acceptance of AI among medical professionals introduces its challenges. Resistance to change and concerns regarding AI's accuracy, its effect on radiologists' roles, and the threat of job displacement can impede its adoption. To overcome these barriers, comprehensive training programs are essential to showcase the value and reliability of AI-assisted diagnostics. Additionally, fostering a cultural shift within healthcare institutions is vital to creating an environment that embraces innovation.

Federated learning has the potential to enhance MRI diagnostic accuracy by aggregating knowledge from diverse datasets while ensuring data privacy. However, achieving consistent performance across healthcare settings requires standardizing data formats, imaging protocols, and AI model specifications. Currently, the healthcare industry lacks uniformity in data collection, storage, and processing, complicating the implementation of universally applicable AI solutions. Efforts toward standardization must address technical data formatting, interoperability, and clinical protocols, necessitating collaboration among healthcare providers, technology developers, and regulatory bodies.

Moreover, integrating AI into medical diagnostics raises significant ethical and legal questions regarding patient consent, data privacy, algorithmic bias, and accountability in the event of diagnostic errors. It is crucial to ensure that AI systems operate within ethical frameworks and legal regulations to maintain public trust. Patients must be informed about how their data is utilized and safeguarded, particularly in federated learning. Rigorous testing and validation must be conducted to ensure equitable and accurate diagnostics across diverse populations. Navigating the regulatory landscape requires a thorough understanding of technology and healthcare law to guarantee compliance with relevant regulations. Despite these challenges, the successful implementation of AI in MRI diagnostics offers efficient, privacy-conscious solutions, paving the way for future advancements in AI diagnostics.

The Transformative Role of AI in ctDNA Testing

By enhancing these assessments' accuracy, sensitivity, and clinical utility, AI enables earlier cancer detection, potentially leading to improved patient outcomes.

Machine learning, a branch of artificial intelligence, employs algorithms to independently derive insights and discern patterns from data, using this understanding to make increasingly informed decisions. It has played a crucial role in developing the Galleri MCED tests. The Galleri test, created by GRAIL, employs AI to examine over one million methylation sites across more than 100,000 genomic regions, identifying abnormal DNA methylation patterns that may signal the presence of cancer.

Initially, a classifier algorithm was trained using sequencing data from over 15,000 participants in the CCGA study conducted between 2016 and 2018. This cohort consisted of 6,670 cancer-free individuals and 8,584 individuals with cancer, with comprehensive records detailing cancer types and any co-morbidities.

The classifier's training began with encoding DNA methylation status into a computer-readable format called "representation." Following this, the algorithm examined methylation patterns from cancer-free participants in the CCGA study, comparing them to those from individuals with cancer, to identify a universal cancer signal, a process known as "learning." This cancer signature is rarely found in individuals confirmed to be cancer-free. The algorithm then assigned a score to each participant to estimate the likelihood of cancer, categorizing these scores into two outcomes: cancer signal detected (test positive) or test negative.

After completing the representation, learning, and scoring steps, the classifier was tested and validated with new, unseen data. If a positive test is indicated, a secondary algorithm is triggered to pinpoint the origin of the cancerous cfDNA fragments, predicting a cancer signal origin (CSO). This approach fosters a continuous learning environment, allowing the classifier to enhance performance by training on increasingly diverse data over time.

AI excels at processing vast datasets and uncovering intricate patterns that may elude human observers. By training AI models on extensive datasets of cfDNA samples from both cancerous and non-cancerous individuals, these algorithms learn to detect subtle molecular signatures associated with various cancer types, enabling highly accurate identification of cancer signals.

Moreover, AI is instrumental in interpreting and classifying detected cancer signals. Once a signal is recognized, AI algorithms analyze specific genetic alteration patterns to predict the tissue of origin, providing essential insights that guide diagnostic procedures and treatment strategies. For example, the Galleri test has shown remarkable success in accurately predicting cancer origins in many positive cases, a feat made possible through AI.

Beyond detection and classification, AI enhances the performance and clinical utility of ctDNA tests. Machine learning techniques optimize test parameters like sensitivity and specificity by analyzing extensive clinical data and refining algorithms accordingly. This iterative refinement process ensures that tests like Galleri stay at the forefront of cancer screening technology, continually improving their ability to detect cancer at the most curable stages.

Additionally, AI can integrate ctDNA test results with other clinical data, including patient demographics, medical history, and imaging findings, to provide a comprehensive cancer risk assessment and guide personalized screening and treatment strategies. This holistic approach aligns with the principles of precision medicine, tailoring cancer care to each patient's unique characteristics and needs.

While integrating AI into ctDNA tests such as Galleri is still in its developmental stages, ongoing research and clinical trials are pushing the boundaries of what is achievable. Large-scale studies, such as the CCGA and PATHFINDER studies, generate invaluable data to train and refine AI models, enhancing their performance and clinical applicability.

In conclusion, integrating AI into ctDNA tests signifies a substantial advancement in cancer detection. By harnessing machine learning and advanced data analysis, these tests achieve unprecedented accuracy in identifying cancer signals, provide insights into the tissue of origin, and pave the way for earlier interventions and improved patient outcomes. As AI technology evolves, its impact on cancer screening and precision medicine will deepen, offering hope for a future where cancer detection and treatment are more effective.

Bright Future: Integrating AI into Early Detection

Artificial Intelligence is revolutionizing medical diagnostics, fundamentally changing how we detect, characterize, and treat diseases. One of its most promising applications lies in enhancing MRI technology for the preventive screening of cancer and other health issues. AI-driven MRI advancements are markedly improving the accuracy, speed, and accessibility of diagnostic imaging, making early detection more practical and effective.

These sophisticated algorithms, trained on extensive datasets of MRI scans, can identify subtle anomalies and patterns that might elude human radiologists, thereby boosting diagnostic precision. For instance, AI can accurately differentiate between benign and malignant lesions, significantly reducing false positives and negatives—a critical capability for early cancer detection, where timely intervention can dramatically improve patient outcomes. Moreover, AI's capacity to analyze vast amounts of data quickly and efficiently streamlines the diagnostic process, resulting in faster results and more timely treatments.

Beyond cancer detection, AI-enhanced MRI plays a crucial role in the early diagnosis of various diseases, including cardiovascular conditions, neurological disorders, and musculoskeletal abnormalities.

As AI continues to evolve and integrate into medical diagnostics, it promises to transform preventive healthcare, enhance early detection, and ultimately improve patient outcomes. The future of AI-powered systemic early detection is indeed bright, with the potential to revolutionize how diseases are detected, managed, and treated, paving the way for effective preventive healthcare

Reducing Costs and Enhancing Equality with AI

CHAPTER NINE

"You're either the one that creates the automation or you're getting automated."
Tom Preston-Werner

How can we make these state-of-the-art systemic early detection tests more affordable and universally accessible?

Early detection has long been a cornerstone in the fight against cancer and other life-threatening diseases. Recent advancements, such as whole-body MRI and blood ctDNA tests, promise to revolutionize preventive care. However, their widespread implementation faces significant challenges concerning accessibility and equity.

Whole-body MRI and ctDNA tests often come with steep costs, creating barriers for individuals from lower socioeconomic backgrounds. This disparity could exacerbate existing health inequalities, leaving those with limited financial resources unable to access these life-saving technologies.

Addressing these issues of accessibility and equity is crucial to ensure that the benefits of innovative technologies reach all segments of society, regardless of socioeconomic status or geographic location. Integrating AI and other technological advancements offers immense potential to enhance these diagnostic tools' automation, efficiency, and affordability, thereby promoting greater equality and accessibility for all.

Smart Phone Adoption: A Case Study

The pursuit of equitable and accessible early detection technologies mirrors the historical evolution of high-tech smartphones. By examining how high-tech cell phones transitioned from exclusive, high-cost items to widely available tools, we can gain insights into the potential advancements in cancer screening.

When commercial cellular phones first emerged in the early 1980s, they were prohibitively expensive. The first cellular phones, such as the Motorola DynaTAC 8000X, were introduced in 1983 and had a retail price of approximately $3,995, equating to over $10,000 today when adjusted for inflation—this high-cost limited access primarily to affluent individuals and businesses.

This exclusivity mirrors the current landscape of whole-body MRI and blood ctDNA tests. For instance, a full-body MRI scan in the United States can range from $650 to >$3,000 without insurance coverage, rendering it inaccessible for many.

Cellular phone adoption experienced a dramatic surge in the mid-1990s to early 2000s, driven by technological advancements and economies of scale that significantly decreased prices and phone sizes. By the late 1990s, the influx of mobile phone models and the entry of various service providers led to competitive pricing, making this technology more accessible. This period of broader adoption and gradual price reductions may foreshadow the future trajectory of diagnostic technologies.

The launch of smartphones in the late 2000s, especially Apple's iPhone in 2007, revolutionized the cellular phone market. Now available for as little as $100, smartphones have evolved into essential tools for daily life, education, and work, achieving near-global ubiquity. This vision of widespread access is what many aspire to for advanced diagnostics like whole-body MRI scans and ctDNA tests—transforming them from luxury items into standard preventive measures in healthcare.

The history of cellular phone adoption provides vital lessons for the future of medical diagnostic technologies. By leveraging strategies from the telecom industry, healthcare stakeholders can strive to make life-saving early detection tools as commonplace and accessible as smartphones. This will improve healthcare outcomes and ensure that advanced diagnostics become a standard resource available to everyone rather than a privilege for the few. Here are some examples of recent advances in reducing MRI cost.

AI-Enabled Low-Cost MRI Scanners

Current superconducting MRI scanners still come with high costs and require specialized environments, keeping them out of reach. These machines are typically found in specialized radiology departments and large imaging centers, which limits their availability at other medical sites. It adds to the hardware costs while reducing mobility and patient comfort due to the required RF-shielded rooms and other high-power consumption. However, AI has a wealth of potential applications in lowering the cost of MRI scanners.

Researchers at the University of Hong Kong recently created a radically simplified ultra-low-field (ULF) MRI scanner that can operate on a standard wall power outlet without needing RF or magnetic shielding. This innovative scanner employs a compact 0.05 Tesla permanent magnet and uses active sensing and AI to mitigate electromagnetic interference (EMI). By deploying EMI sensing coils around the scanner and implementing a deep learning method, they can directly predict EMI-free nuclear magnetic resonance signals from the acquired data.

Moreover, the team developed a data-driven deep-learning image formation method to enhance image quality and reduce scan time. This method integrates image reconstruction with three-dimensional multiscale super-resolution and leverages homogeneous human anatomy and image contrasts available in large-scale, high-field, high-resolution MRI data. Their partial Fourier super-resolution (PF-SR) method combines image reconstruction and super-resolution techniques. The PF-SR model, which includes multiscale feature extraction, spatial attention, and reconstruction functions, was experimentally validated by comparing 0.055 T brain images to 3 T images from the same subjects. Typically involving 3D encoding with k-space partial Fourier sampling, this approach advanced the quality of 0.05 T MRI images by effectively suppressing artifacts and noise while increasing spatial resolution. The PF-SR method produced isotropic 1-mm resolution, significantly enhancing the clarity of 0.05 T images.

This lower-power, AI-assisted MRI machine is more affordable to manufacture and operate, more comfortable and quieter for patients, and produces images as clear and detailed as those from high-power devices currently used in clinical settings. The AI-enabled lower-power MRI machine represents a potential revolution in MRI technology, offering a widely accessible, economical point-of-care imaging tool.

AI-Enabled Faster MRI Scanning

AI-enabled rapid MRI scanning is an innovative technique designed to reduce MRI scan times while ensuring high diagnostic quality.

Integrating AI into MRI technology also addresses the issue of prolonged scan times, which can impede widespread use in preventive screenings. Traditional MRI scans often take a long time and can be uncomfortable for patients, limiting their practicality for routine assessments. However, AI technologies, including deep learning algorithms, can significantly shorten MRI scan durations without sacrificing image quality. By acquiring only a fraction of the data typically needed for a complete MRI scan and employing AI to reconstruct the missing information, scan times can be reduced by as much as 83%. This advancement enhances patient comfort and increases the accessibility and affordability of MRI screenings. For example, the fastMRI initiative by NYU and Meta AI has proven capable of cutting scan times by 75% while maintaining diagnostic accuracy, making routine MRI screenings more feasible, particularly for high-risk individuals and those with a family history of cancer.

In recent decades, considerable research has focused on accelerating MRI through advanced data sampling and reconstruction techniques. These approaches often utilize rapid acquisition schemes that deviate from the classical Nyquist-sampling criterion, a method known as undersampling. While this can introduce image-domain artifacts, well-designed reconstruction techniques are vital for preserving clinical-quality images. Deep learning (DL) methods have recently achieved state-of-the-art results in this domain, enabling high acceleration with exceptional reconstruction quality. Their success stems from the ability to learn image priors in a data-driven manner, contrasting with the hand-crafted techniques used in compressed sensing and dictionary learning.

Physics-guided unrolled neural networks effectively combine the advantages of DL-based artifact removal with data consistency blocks, integrating a physics-based imaging system model. Extensive research has demonstrated the benefits of DL in reconstructing 2D MRI scans, and attention has recently shifted towards using DL to accelerate higher-dimensional MRI scans, such as dynamic MRI.

Numerous studies have proposed techniques to develop DL models while addressing data-related challenges. One such framework for dynamic MRI reconstruction, self-supervised collaborative learning (SelcCoLearn), operates without relying on ground truth data. This framework divides undersampled k-space measurements into two datasets, inputs for two parallel neural networks with identical architectures but different weights. A co-training loss ensures consistency between the predictions of both networks. Experiments using cardiac data have shown that SelcCoLearn produces high-quality reconstructions of dynamic MRI data.

Deep learning-based methods have also been introduced for denoising low-SNR diffusion-weighted images (DWI) of rectal cancer acquired at high b-values, utilizing low b-value DWI images as guidance. Blind tests conducted by radiologists reveal that these methods facilitate an eight-fold acceleration in scan time.

Ezra has made significant strides in reducing scanning time through the integration of AI. Their proprietary technology, Ezra Flash, has received FDA clearance and enhances MR image quality, enabling shorter scan times and reduced MRI costs. The company aims to launch 30-minute full-body MRI scans, leveraging this technology. Ezra Flash was trained on the company's proprietary longitudinal MRI dataset, which includes hundreds of thousands of MR images from patients and healthy individuals. The AI was designed to recognize critical elements in MRI scans essential for producing complete and accurate images. A panel of radiologists has validated the software's performance, confirming its effectiveness. This multi-step validation process has allowed Ezra to improve image quality in high-speed MRI scans that challenge current standards of care. Previously, the Ezra Full Body MRI took one hour and cost $1,950; it is now available as a 30-minute scan for $1,350, representing a 30% cost reduction. Ezra aims to offer a 15-minute full-body MRI scan for $500 in the near future.

In summary, AI-enabled faster MRI scanning employs machine learning to reconstruct diagnostic images from undersampled data and reduce scan times while preserving imaging quality, thus significantly decreasing MRI scan costs.

MRI Automation with AI

Over the past decade, AI has profoundly influenced various fields, including science, engineering, informatics, finance, and transportation. More recently, it has opened up new avenues to improve the quality and efficiency of patient care. Given that the initial breakthroughs in deep learning focused on image perception, interpretation, and analysis, it is no surprise that this technology has driven significant advancements in medical imaging. For example, deep learning techniques have achieved state-of-the-art image formation, analysis, pathology detection, and protocol planning outcomes.

AI-assisted image analysis can streamline the interpretation of whole-body MRI scans, alleviating the workload of radiologists and facilitating more efficient and accurate diagnoses. AI algorithms can be trained to identify subtle abnormalities and patterns that may be difficult for human experts to detect, potentially improving the sensitivity and specificity of early disease detection.

AI techniques have recently reached state-of-the-art performance in the automated segmentation of structures and pathologies, including brain tumors and abdominal tissues/organs. However, developing effective AI methods requires large training datasets, which are often scarce due to the high costs associated with data labeling. Furthermore, utilizing off-label datasets can introduce bias. Researchers have investigated the advantages of pre-training segmentation networks on varied datasets for different tasks to address these challenges.

Automated scan prescription is an emerging AI application with significant potential for optimizing clinical workflows. Traditionally, MRI scans necessitate labor-intensive manual prescriptions reliant on human expertise. Innovative techniques have been introduced to automate this process, including an automatic field-of-view prescription system that utilizes an intra-stack attention neural network. This advanced system surpasses standard CNN models and generates prescriptions that closely align with those created by radiologists. Validated with pediatric pelvic and abdominal images, this method has shown clinically acceptable results alongside rapid inference times.

Recent advancements in AI have significantly transformed MRI workflows, impacting every stage of the imaging process—from protocol planning and data acquisition to image reconstruction, quantitative parameter mapping, and automated segmentation. AI's influence extends to automated diagnosis and prognosis, facilitating the detection conditions such as breast and prostate cancer from MRI scans and enabling fault detection in health management systems. These AI methods have achieved state-of-the-art outcomes in lesion detection and classification.

AI has revolutionized numerous aspects of MRI, from accelerating scan times to improving image reconstruction and automated analysis. Deep learning models can intelligently reconstruct high-quality diagnostic images from undersampled MRI data, reducing scan times by up to 75% while maintaining accuracy. This advancement not only enhances patient comfort but also increases accessibility and throughput. AI techniques have streamlined workflows, enabling automated scan planning, organ segmentation, lesion detection, and quantitative analysis, thereby augmenting the capabilities of radiologists. Furthermore, AI is being harnessed for advanced applications, including image synthesis, parameter mapping, and the integration of multimodal data, pushing MRI technology's boundaries. Initiatives like fastMRI have publicly made AI models and datasets available, fostering collaboration and driving innovation.

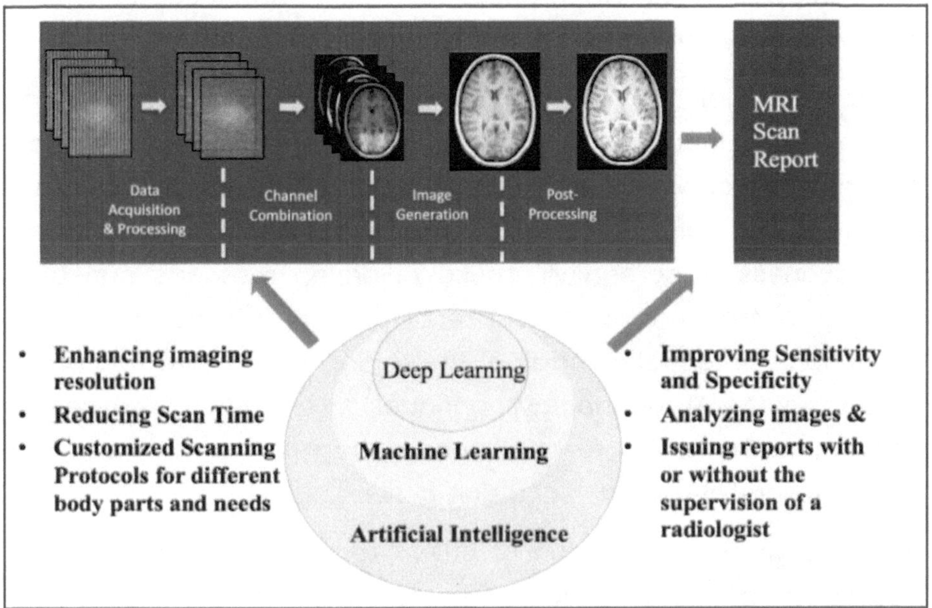

As the field continues to evolve, AI promises to optimize MRI acquisition, reconstruction, and interpretation, ultimately enhancing diagnostic precision and improving patient care at low costs.

Reducing Blood ctDNA Test Costs with AI

ctDNA tests have emerged as a robust early cancer detection and monitoring tool. However, their widespread adoption has been hindered by high costs.

Automation is pivotal in reducing costs by minimizing human intervention and boosting efficiency. For ctDNA tests, automating sample preparation, DNA extraction, and analysis can significantly lessen hands-on time and the risk of human error. Sophisticated robotic liquid handling systems and automated DNA extraction platforms now enable high-throughput processing with minimal human involvement.

This not only cuts labor costs but also enhances the reproducibility and reliability of test results.

Artificial intelligence and machine learning further drive cost reductions by increasing the sensitivity and specificity of mutation detection. AI-powered analysis can potentially decrease the need for repeat testing, thereby improving the overall cost-effectiveness of screening. These AI-driven methods can also identify patterns and biomarkers that may escape human detection, potentially leading to earlier and more accurate diagnoses. As AI technology continues to evolve, it promises to streamline the ctDNA testing process, from sample handling to data interpretation, further cutting costs.

With the growing adoption of ctDNA tests, economies of scale contribute to cost reductions. A more extensive user base allows fixed equipment, R&D, and infrastructure costs to be distributed across more tests, lowering the per-test expense. Bulk purchasing of sequencing reagents and materials can lead to significant savings. Moreover, increased test volume enables laboratories to optimize workflows and resource allocation, driving costs down further. Integrating these tests into routine clinical practice could standardize protocols across healthcare systems, enhancing efficiency and reducing costs.

The synergy of automation, AI, and economies of scale presents a promising avenue for lowering ctDNA test costs. As these technologies advance and gain wider adoption, ctDNA tests will likely become more affordable and accessible, potentially revolutionizing early cancer detection and improving patient outcomes.

Envisioning a Future of Universal Accessibility for Systemic Early Detection

AI is poised to make advanced early detection tests like whole-body MRI and ctDNA tests universally accessible. As we envision a future where these powerful diagnostic tools are widely available,

AI emerges as a critical enabler, addressing current limitations and opening new possibilities for early disease detection and personalized medicine. AI has the potential to significantly improve the efficiency of these procedures, reduce costs, and enhance diagnostic accuracy. For whole-body MRI, AI algorithms can optimize scan protocols and automated image analysis, while in ctDNA tests, AI can streamline DNA sequencing and improve mutation and methylation detection accuracy.

The integration of AI into these diagnostic tools offers the promise of personalized screening and early cancer detection. By analyzing vast amounts of data, including genetic information, lifestyle factors, and imaging data, AI algorithms can help identify individuals who would benefit most from whole-body MRI or ctDNA screening. This personalized approach could optimize resource allocation, ensuring these advanced diagnostic tools are used most effectively. Furthermore, AI can facilitate the integration of whole-body MRI and ctDNA tests into telemedicine platforms, allowing for remote interpretation of results and making these technologies accessible even in areas without specialized radiologists or genetic counselors.

One of the most potent aspects of AI is its ability to learn and improve over time. As more data is collected from whole-body MRI scans and ctDNA tests, AI algorithms can continuously refine their accuracy and efficiency, potentially leading to new biomarkers or imaging features associated with various diseases. This continuous improvement and AI's ability to support general radiologists and genetic counselors can help address the shortage of specialists that currently limits the widespread adoption of these advanced diagnostic tools.

While AI offers tremendous potential, its integration into early detection also raises important ethical considerations. Ensuring the privacy and security of patient data, maintaining transparency in AI decision-making processes, and addressing potential biases in AI algorithms are crucial challenges that must be addressed. As we move towards a future of universal accessibility for whole-body MRI and ctDNA tests, the integration of AI must be guided by principles of equity, transparency, and patient-centered care. With thoughtful implementation, AI has the potential to democratize access to advanced diagnostics, leading to earlier disease detection, more personalized intervention strategies, and, ultimately, better health and well-being for populations worldwide.

In conclusion, the future of whole-body MRI and ctDNA tests holds tremendous promise for revolutionizing proactive cancer care and healthcare.

Through the synergistic effects of technological development, automation, AI, and economies of scale, we can envision a world where these AI-powered diagnostic tools are universally accessible.

PART III

The Guide

Taking Action to Catch Most Cancers Early and Save Lives

The Dawn of a New Era of Systemic Early Detection .

The Dawn of a New Era of Systemic Early Detection

CHAPTER TEN

"Take care of your body. It's the only place you have to live in."
Jim Rohan

What is the most effective and practical approach to defeating cancer?

The answer lies in systemic early detection throughout the entire body to catch most cancers at their early, curable stages. This conclusion is grounded in our profound understanding and thorough assessment of cancer treatment, prevention, and screening advancements.

This chapter will explore why systemic early detection is the most effective and practical approach to defeating cancer and how these cutting-edge tests can be adopted in a timely manner.

Here, let's take a look at the following data, presenting the current dire status of cancer care:

In the United States:

- In 2023, an estimated 1,958,310 new cancer cases and 609,820 cancer deaths are projected to occur.

- In 2024, an estimated 2,001,140 new cancer cases and 611,720 cancer deaths are projected.

Globally:

- In 2022, there were an estimated 19.3 million new cancer cases and 10 million cancer deaths worldwide.

- The global cancer burden is projected to grow to 29.4 million new cases and 16.8 million deaths by 2040 due to population growth and aging.

- The total number of cancer deaths increased by 75% between 1990-2019, likely due to population growth and aging.

Amid the dire statistics, one encouraging sign is the decline in the cancer mortality rate in the US (despite the overall increase in total mortality), primarily due to cancer prevention and early detection. While cancer prevention and early detection through screening are crucial in reducing the burden of cancer, they remain severely underfunded and underappreciated compared to cancer treatment.

The American Cancer Society estimates that less than 10% of its budget is allocated to prevention and early detection programs. Here are some facts:

- Approximately 60% of cancers are still diagnosed at an advanced stage, where treatment is often ineffective and costly.

- The 5-year relative survival rate for localized cancers is 90%, compared to less than 25% for cancers diagnosed at a distant stage, across most cancer types.

- It is estimated that 30-50% of cancer cases could be prevented through lifestyle changes and adherence to current early detection recommendations.

Despite the clear benefits of cancer prevention and early detection, funding remains disproportionately low compared to treatment for late-stage cancers that only marginally extend life. Redirecting resources towards prevention and screening could significantly reduce cancer burden and healthcare costs.

So why are cancer prevention and early detection so underfunded? Here are several key factors contributing to the significant funding gap between cancer treatment and early detection/prevention:

Immediate vs. Long-Term Impact: Cancer treatment offers an immediate and visible impact on patients' lives, making it a more compelling cause for funding. In contrast, the benefits of prevention and screening efforts, though substantial in the long run, are not as readily apparent in the short term.

Advocacy and Lobbying: Pharmaceutical companies, medical professionals, and patient advocacy groups have a strong lobbying presence, advocating for increased funding for cancer treatment research and drug development. Prevention and screening efforts often lack such powerful advocacy voices.

Profit Incentives: There is a significant financial incentive for pharmaceutical companies to invest in developing new cancer treatments, as they can generate substantial profits from successful drugs. Prevention and screening efforts, which often involve lifestyle changes, screening, and public health initiatives, offer less potential for direct financial gain.

Complexity of Prevention and Screening: Cancer prevention and screening involves tackling a wide range of factors, including lifestyle, environmental exposures, and socioeconomic determinants of health. This complexity makes it challenging to develop and implement effective prevention strategies, which can discourage funding.

Despite the clear advantages of cancer prevention and early detection in reducing the overall burden of the disease and associated healthcare costs, funding disparity persists due to these combined factors. Addressing this gap will require a concerted effort to raise awareness, advocate for prevention initiatives, and demonstrate preventive measures' long-term impact and cost-effectiveness.

As detailed in earlier chapters, advanced-stage cancers remain largely incurable. Cancer prevention faces the insurmountable obstacle of aging, the biggest yet non-modifiable risk factor. Therefore, cancer screening and early detection become the most effective and feasible approaches to defeating cancer.

The Need for Systemic Early Detection

The call for a transformative shift resonates globally within healthcare institutions and research facilities. We need a paradigm shift—a seismic move away from the reactive, symptom-driven approach that has dominated cancer management for decades. Instead, a proactive stance is essential, leveraging the full potential of technology and innovation to detect cancer at its earliest, most curable stages.

Proactive screening is pivotal in ushering in a new era of cancer care, where the disease is identified before symptoms appear. By systematically applying tests and assessments to asymptomatic individuals, we can detect cancer in its nascent stages or even identify precancerous conditions before they progress into full-blown malignancies. The benefits of this approach are evident: enhanced treatment effectiveness, improved survival rates, reduced treatment-related morbidity, and lower healthcare costs—a true paradigm shift in the battle against cancer.

The stark reality of cancer's impact on humanity calls for action, demanding a multifaceted response. Technological innovation must work in tandem with policy reform and public education, fostering an environment where routine screenings become standard practice and early symptoms are promptly recognized and addressed.

Therefore, shifting our focus from treatment to early detection is imperative. Systemic early detection of most types of cancer, not a cure, is the crucial factor in conquering this disease.

The Hope: Emerging Systemic Early Detection with a Single Test

Addressing Huge Gaps in Cancer Screening

Currently, cancer screening and early detection are recommended for only two types of cancer (colorectal and lung) in men and four types of cancer in women (including breast and cervical). While better implementation of existing single-site cancer screening tests is essential, it remains insufficient, leaving significant gaps. There is an urgent need for new cancer screening technologies and tests.

Fortunately, two sophisticated systemic early detection technologies have emerged, detailed in earlier chapters and summarized here.

Whole-Body MRI: Revealing the Black Box

Whole-body MRI scans offer a comprehensive, non-invasive method for detecting cancer and other abnormalities throughout the body. Unlike traditional imaging techniques that rely on ionizing radiation, MRI uses magnetic resonance imaging, providing a safer option for repeated use.

For years, MRI has been a cornerstone in cancer diagnostics. Recent advancements in MRI technology have elevated its capabilities to unprecedented levels, enabling higher-resolution imaging. These improvements allow healthcare professionals to detect tumors at their earliest stages, a previously unattainable precision level. Whole-body MRI can identify tumors before they spread, offering several key advantages:

- Comprehensive Screening: Whole-body MRI can detect a diverse range of cancers, from those in the brain and spine to those in the chest, abdomen, and pelvis.

- Early Detection: With highly sensitivity, MRI can unveil tumors at their earliest stages, even before symptoms appear, providing a valuable window for curable treatment.

- Safe and Non-Invasive: The procedure is gentle and free from the risks associated with invasive or harmful radiation-based imaging methods.

Blood ctDNA Tests: Sensing the Hidden Signals

Beyond imaging, cutting-edge circulating tumor DNA (ctDNA) tests for Multi-Cancer Early Detection (MCED) can revolutionize cancer screening. These tests analyze DNA shed by tumors into the bloodstream, offering a minimally invasive option for early detection of most cancer types, including pancreatic and ovarian cancer without existing screening tests, with a single test. ctDNA tests represent a cutting-edge cancer detection and monitoring approach, offering a minimally invasive method to identify the disease's presence. The advantages of ctDNA tests include:

- Early Detection: For most cancer types with a single blood test. These tests can detect cancer at an early stage, sometimes even before tumors are visible through imaging, allowing for early, curable intervention.

- Minimally Invasive: As a simple blood test, ctDNA testing reduces the risk and discomfort associated with traditional biopsy or invasive methods.

Integration of Systemic Detection Technology with AI

In an era of exponential data growth, the sheer volume of information necessary to unlock cancer's secrets has surpassed human capabilities. Enter AI, our formidable ally in this battle. These advanced algorithms are adept at detecting subtle patterns and anomalies in medical images, genetic data, and patient records—nuances that might escape even the most skilled human analysts. AI-driven whole-body MRI and ctDNA tests are capable of detecting most cancer types at early, curable stages with a single test.

Benefits of Cancer Screening and Early Detection

A 2023 study published in BMC Health Services Research by teams from the University of Chicago and the University of Michigan used a mathematical model to evaluate the impact of four cancer screenings recommended by the US Preventive Services Task Force (USPSTF). The USPSTF assesses evidence around preventive medical services and issues recommendations using letter grades. Since 2010, the Affordable Care Act has mandated that screenings and services with "A" or "B" grades be covered by most insurance plans at no cost to the patient.

"Screenings for breast, colorectal, cervical, and lung cancer have saved millions of life years, yet their full potential is still unmet," remarked A. Mark Fendrick, MD, senior author of the study and a professor of internal medicine and public health at U-M. "Many Americans who could benefit from early detection of these cancers remain unscreened, even though these tests are typically available without out-of-pocket costs for those with health insurance." Fendrick directs the U-M Center for Value-Based Insurance Design.

It is estimated that preventive cancer screenings in the past 25 years have granted Americans at least 12 million additional years of life. This equates to a staggering $6.5 trillion in economic impact, thanks to early detection of breast, colon, cervical, and lung cancers in high-risk adults. This figure does not even account for the medical cost savings from treating cancer at an earlier stage rather than a later one.

The findings highlight the need to encourage more people to undergo recommended cancer screenings and innovate new methods for detecting other cancers.

"Earlier detection is key to addressing late-stage cancer costs," wrote Josh Ofman, M.D., President of Grail. He emphasized that treatment costs escalate with the advancement of cancer stages. For instance, treating metastatic cancers can be up to seven times more expensive than treating early-stage cancers. Specifically, early-stage cervical cancer treatment costs around $37,000, while advanced-stage treatment can soar to $282,000.

Other research has demonstrated that a cancer diagnosis brings substantial indirect costs, such as reduced productivity, increased absenteeism, and changes in employment status for both patients and caregivers. A recent study revealed that productivity loss and indirect costs are significantly higher for patients diagnosed with late-stage cancer compared to early-stage cancer.

The individual impact quickly accumulates to a massive system-wide burden. Within the next decade, cancer costs are projected to exceed $245 billion annually, with the highest expenses associated with late-stage diagnoses. However, there is a significant opportunity for improvement. A recent analysis estimated that early diagnosis across 19 cancers could result in $26 billion in cost savings, approximately 17% of direct treatment costs. Additionally, incorporating MCED (multi-cancer early detection) tests into standard care is highly cost-effective, reducing cancer treatment costs by over $5,000 per patient and improving long-term health outcomes.

We must expand our screening capabilities to reduce cancer mortality and costs further. Currently, screenings are available for only three types of cancer in women, two in men, with an additional screening for heavy smokers. We need to move beyond this limited paradigm and implement broader screening strategies to detect cancers early, when outcomes are better, quality of life is improved, and costs are lower.

Enacting the Transformation

Resources and Efforts Required for Systemic Early Detection

In the epic battle against cancer, early detection shines as a beacon of hope, guiding us towards a future where late-stage diagnoses become a thing of the past.

Achieving this future demands unwavering commitment and collective action. Transforming early cancer detection is an ambitious endeavor, requiring the mobilization of resources and coordinated efforts across multiple dimensions.

A nationwide transformation is essential—a metamorphosis of facilities and technology. Healthcare institutions are reimagined and expanded to embrace a new era of cancer screening. State-of-the-art MRI machines are being installed, equipped for efficient whole-body scans, their powerful magnets poised to explore the depths of the human body.

A new generation of healthcare professionals is crucial. Radiologists refine their skills, learning to interpret whole-body MRI scans with precision, their eyes trained to detect even the faintest signs of malignancy. Technicians master the intricate protocols of these advanced scans, ensuring patient safety and comfort while maximizing efficiency.

In boardrooms and legislative chambers, rigorous economic analyses are underway. Cost-effectiveness studies weigh the investment in screening against the potential healthcare savings from earlier cancer intervention. Negotiations with insurance companies and government agencies are ongoing, forging reimbursement frameworks to make widespread access to whole-body MRI screening a reality.

Envision a harmonious collaboration: governments, non-profits, and private entities unite to form public-private partnerships that transcend traditional boundaries. This collective mission aims to pool resources, eliminate redundancies, and ensure early detection benefits reach every corner of the nation.

As this visionary program unfolds, a crucial element emerges: the public health strategy. Expert panels meticulously craft guidelines dictating who should be screened, how often, and under what conditions, balancing risk factors and potential benefits. Concurrently, a nationwide public education campaign informs and empowers the populace. Through various channels, people are educated about early detection's promise, dispelling myths, and fostering a culture of proactive health management.

In the digital realm, a fortress of data security is essential. Within this secure environment, researchers diligently collect and analyze screening data, refine protocols, improve outcomes, and adapt strategies as new evidence emerges.

The Winding Road to Regulatory Approval

FDA approval is critical to market a new test. The FDA plays a pivotal role in this process through its rigorous approval protocols for new cancer screening and early detection tests. The FDA's mandate focuses on ensuring that new tests are both safe and effective before being available to the public. This involves a comprehensive review process assessing the clinical utility of the tests and the risks they might pose to patients.

Pre-Market Approval Process. Most new cancer screening tests, such as ctDNA, undergo the Pre-Market Approval (PMA) process— the FDA's most stringent regulatory pathway. This process necessitates the manufacturer to submit substantial data, including clinical trial results demonstrating the test's efficacy and safety. The approval process includes:

a. Scientific Validity. The test must be scientifically valid, effectively measuring or detecting the condition it claims to, such as the presence of cancerous cells or markers.

b. Clinical Validity. The test must demonstrate clinical validity and accurately and reliably identify or predict cancer risk in a general population. This involves extensive clinical trials or well-designed studies providing robust data on sensitivity (the ability to correctly identify those with the disease), specificity (the ability to correctly identify those without the disease), and predictive values (how well the test predicts the presence or absence of the disease).

c. Clinical Utility. The test must show clinical utility, meaning its use leads to improved clinical outcomes. This implies that the test should contribute to better decision-making in clinical practice, leading to more effective prevention, diagnosis, or treatment of cancer. Demonstrating the ability of cancer screening tests to reduce cancer death rates in a population presents significant challenges due to the nature of cancer and the complexities of conducting large-scale randomized controlled trials (RCTs). RCTs are the gold standard for assessing screening efficacy—comparing outcomes between a screened population and an unscreened control group. RCTs often require large numbers of participants and multi-year follow-ups, complicating logistics and increasing costs. Longitudinal studies over many years or decades are required to demonstrate a statistically significant reduction in mortality, involving considerable time, effort, and funding.

d. Risk-Benefit Analysis. The FDA conducts a risk-benefit analysis to determine if the benefits of the test for the intended population outweigh the risks. This analysis considers potential harms from false positives (unnecessary worry and invasive follow-up procedures) and false negatives (missed cancers). The delicate ethical balance between the potential benefits of early cancer detection and the harms caused by overdiagnosis and overtreatment necessitates careful communication of the risks and benefits of screening to the public.

Impact of Regulatory Delays: A Delicate Balance

Maintaining a delicate balance in healthcare innovation is crucial—between the urgency of life-saving advancements and the necessity for thorough scrutiny. Regulatory delays in the approval process carry profound implications, acting as a double-edged sword for those tirelessly pushing the boundaries of medical science.

On one side, the promise of innovative tests that could save countless lives is tantalizing yet hindered by the intricate web of regulations. Each passing day leaves lives hanging in the balance, underscoring the urgent need for progress.

Conversely, a voice of reason calls for caution and meticulous review. This rigorous vetting process mitigates potential harm, ensuring that tests released to the public are safe, effective, and worthy of their trust.

Delays in approval can have significant repercussions. On one hand, they may postpone the availability of life-saving innovative tests. On the other, thorough reviews are crucial to prevent the dissemination of inadequately vetted tests that could cause harm.

Laboratory-Developled Test: Direct to Consumers

Laboratory-developed tests (LDTs) are essential in modern diagnostic laboratories, offering customized and innovative solutions for various medical conditions, including genetic testing and cancer screening. The direct-to-consumer (DTC) model allows these tests to be marketed and sold directly to the public without healthcare provider intermediation.

LDTs are in vitro diagnostic tests designed, manufactured, and used within a single laboratory, addressing specific clinical needs unmet by commercially available tests. Traditionally, healthcare providers interpret these test results in the patient's overall health context. However, the DTC model bypasses this pathway, enabling individuals to order tests and receive results directly, often via online platforms.

Regulatory oversight of LDTs, especially those marketed directly to consumers, varies significantly across jurisdictions. This framework is primarily governed by the FDA and the Centers for Medicare & Medicaid Services (CMS) under the Clinical Laboratory Improvement Amendments (CLIA) in the United States.

Historically, the FDA has exercised enforcement discretion over LDTs, meaning it has not actively regulated these tests as stringently as other in vitro diagnostic devices. This approach has fostered innovation and rapid development within clinical laboratories. In recent years, the FDA has raised concerns about the safety, efficacy, and clinical validity of LDTs, particularly those marketed directly to consumers. The agency has highlighted the need for more comprehensive regulatory oversight to ensure these tests are reliable and provide consumers with accurate information.

The CMS adheres to CLIA regulations. Under CLIA, laboratories conducting LDTs must meet stringent quality standards to ensure test results' accuracy, reliability, and timeliness. CLIA certification is mandatory for any laboratory performing clinical tests, including those offering DTC services. While CLIA ensures the quality of laboratory processes, it does not address the clinical validity or utility of the tests, which are crucial for consumer protection in the DTC market.

One of the primary challenges in regulating DTC LDTs is ensuring their clinical validity and utility. Clinical validity refers to a test's ability to accurately and reliably predict the presence of a condition. In contrast, clinical utility pertains to the test's usefulness in clinical decision-making and patient outcomes. Without the guidance of healthcare professionals, consumers may misinterpret test results, leading to unnecessary anxiety, inappropriate medical decisions, or a false sense of security. Clear, understandable information and appropriate counseling are essential in the DTC model. The marketing of DTC LDTs must be truthful and not misleading; regulatory bodies must ensure companies do not overstate their tests' capabilities or benefits, which could mislead consumers about the test's accuracy and clinical relevance.

The direct-to-consumer model for laboratory-developed tests, including genetic and cancer screening tests, presents both opportunities and challenges. While it can empower consumers with valuable health information, it raises significant regulatory, ethical, and safety concerns. As the use of DTC LDTs continues to grow, it is essential for regulatory bodies to establish and enforce comprehensive frameworks that ensure the safety, reliability, and clinical validity of these tests.

For example, the Galleri MCED test, which has not yet been approved by the FDA, has been marketed directly to consumers as an innovative LDT based on positive clinical trial data.

510(k) Clearance for Medical Device

For tests that are modifications of already approved devices or substantially equivalent to an existing test, such as software upgrades to MRI scanners for whole-body MRI scans, the 510(k) clearance pathway may be utilized.

This process requires the new device to be "substantially equivalent" in terms of safety and effectiveness to an already approved device. It is generally less rigorous than the PMA process but still requires detailed evidence and data. This involves:

a. Substantial Equivalence: The manufacturer must demonstrate that the new test is substantially equivalent to an already FDA-approved test in terms of safety and effectiveness.

b. Supporting Data: Supporting data might include comparative studies against the predicate device, literature reviews, and sometimes clinical data, depending on the extent of changes from the original device.

The FDA approval process for cancer screening tests is designed to evaluate their safety, effectiveness, and utility before market introduction. This thorough assessment ensures that cancer screening tests provide reliable, useful, and safe information for early cancer detection and management, safeguarding public health.

Ezra Flash, an innovative whole-body MRI service, recently achieved a significant milestone by receiving the FDA's 510(k) clearance. This clearance validates the safety and efficacy of Ezra Flash's imaging technology, permitting its use and marketing in clinical settings across the United States. The 510(k) process demonstrates that a medical device is as safe and effective as an existing one, confirming that Ezra Flash meets regulatory standards. This achievement marks a critical step toward making advanced medical imaging more accessible and affordable. By leveraging artificial intelligence, the company enhances diagnostic accuracy and efficiency. Additionally, offering its services at a lower cost compared to traditional MRI scans aims to make routine health screenings more affordable and accessible, especially for individuals at higher risk for cancer. The FDA's clearance underscores the service's safety and clinical effectiveness, allowing Ezra to reach a broader audience and potentially revolutionize early cancer detection and healthcare outcomes.

Given the tremendous potential of these emerging systemic early detection tests, it is imperative to make utmost efforts to develop, adopt, and implement these life-saving technologies promptly. This will lead to a new era where the burden of cancer is significantly reduced, paving the way for a healthier, more equitable society.

The Necessity of Preventive Care

Current healthcare, also known as "sick care," has largely been reactive, concentrating on treating symptoms and managing diseases only after they become apparent and often severe. This "sick care" model, while effective in acute situations, falls short for chronic diseases, where early intervention can drastically alter outcomes. A new paradigm—personalized preventive healthcare—is emerging, focusing on early detection, prevention, and customized treatment strategies.

Current "Sick Care" Model

The prevalent healthcare model operates reactively—patients typically seek medical help only after symptoms manifest. While this approach is necessary for acute and emergency care, it has significant drawbacks when applied to chronic diseases:

- **Late Diagnosis and Ineffective Treatment:** Chronic diseases such as diabetes, heart disease, and cancer often progress silently. When symptoms prompt a doctor's visit, the condition may have advanced to a stage where treatment options are limited and less effective.

- **Higher Healthcare Costs:** Late-stage treatments are often more invasive and expensive.

- **Poorer Outcomes:** Patients diagnosed at later stages of chronic diseases often face poorer prognoses. This is particularly evident in diseases like cancer, where early detection can significantly improve survival rates.

Preventive Healthcare Model

Personalized preventive healthcare represents a paradigm shift towards anticipating and preventing illness before it occurs. This model leverages advancements in imaging, genomics, biotechnology, and data analytics to tailor prevention and treatment plans to individual patients. Key aspects include:

- **Early Detection and Regular Monitoring:** Regular health screenings and predictive analytics can identify risk factors and early lesions.

- **Early Intervention:** Personalized plans can include recommendations for surgery for precancerous lesions, diet, exercise, and stress management tailored to individual needs. Such interventions can significantly reduce the likelihood of developing chronic conditions.

- **Cost-Effectiveness:** Preventing or managing chronic diseases early is generally more cost-effective than treating advanced stages. This not only reduces direct healthcare costs, but also indirect costs related to loss of productivity and long-term care needs.

The transition from sick care to personalized preventive healthcare offers several advantages. Primarily, it promotes a higher quality of life through early intervention and reduces the burden of chronic diseases on individuals and healthcare systems. While the initial costs of integrating advanced technologies and conducting regular screenings might be high, the long-term savings and health benefits are substantial.

Personalized preventive healthcare provides a promising alternative to the traditional reactive sick care model, particularly for managing chronic diseases. By focusing on early detection, tailored interventions, and regular monitoring, this approach can improve health outcomes, reduce healthcare costs, and enhance quality of life.

Highest Health Care Expenditure with Lowest Life Expectancy in OECD Countries

The United States, with its advanced hospitals and healthcare facilities, has been at the forefront of modern medicine and medical technology. Most healthcare resources in the US are directed toward treating patients with severe diseases. Particularly, a substantial portion of cancer care costs is dedicated to end-of-life care. This expenditure is driven by intensive treatments, hospitalizations, and aggressive medical interventions during the terminal stages of cancer, placing significant financial, labor, and psychological burdens on healthcare systems, patients, and their families.

"Despite spending far more on healthcare than other countries, the US does not achieve better outcomes. Life expectancy and other health metrics in the US are worse compared to other parts of the world," wrote Jeff Lagasse in Healthcare Finance. According to a recent report from the Commonwealth Fund (2023), the US spent 17.8% of its GDP on healthcare, nearly double the average of the 38 OECD (Organization for Economic Co-operation and Development) member countries (2022 OECD Health Statistics). Health spending per person in the US was nearly twice as high as in Germany and four times higher than in South Korea. Yet, the US has the lowest life expectancy, the highest death rates for avoidable or treatable conditions, and the highest rate of multiple chronic conditions, with an obesity rate almost twice the OECD average. The diagram illustrates the health expenditure as a percentage of GDP and per capita, alongside life expectancy in the USA and several representative countries.

Thus, the United States has the best "sick-care" system globally on a fee-for-service basis, but this has not translated into better health outcomes for its people.

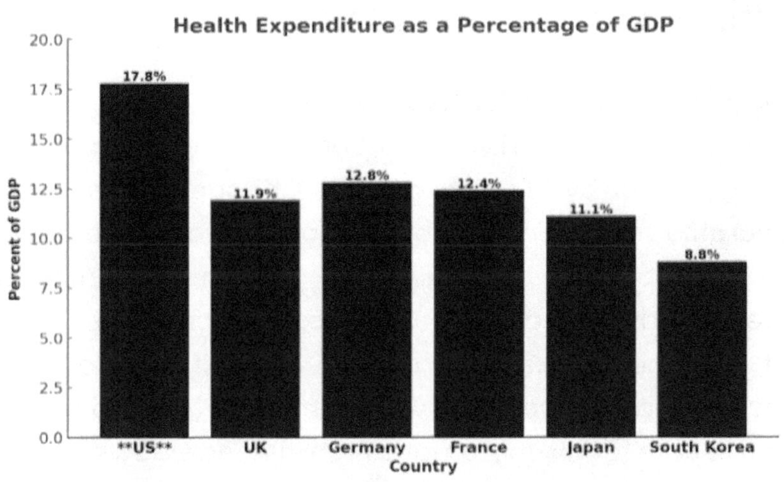

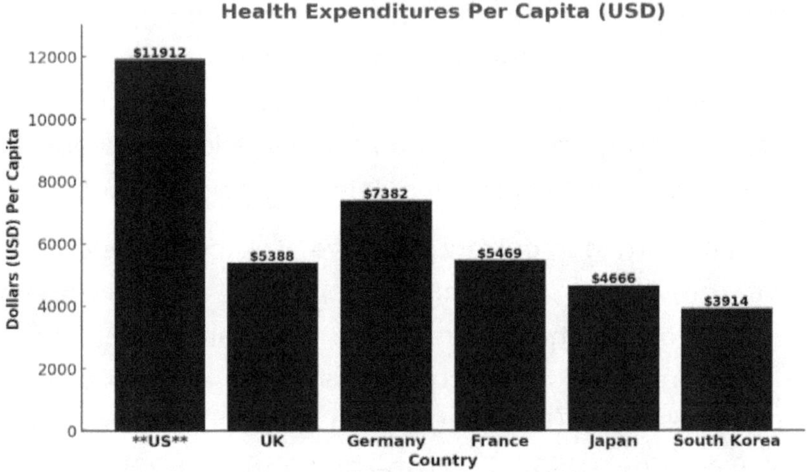

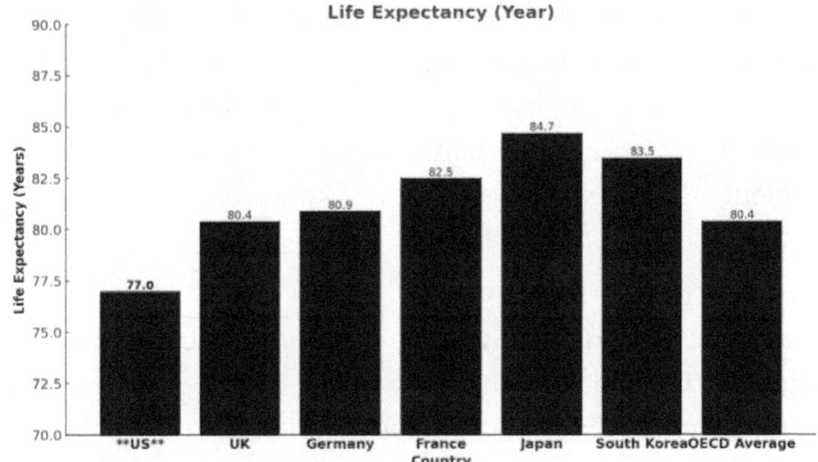

Source: OECD Health Statistics 2022

Prioritizing Systemic Early Detection:

Three Tiers of Anti-Cancer Strategies

Systemic early detection is the most effective, crucial approach to defeating cancer by identifying tumors throughout the body at early, curable stages. Early detection not only saves lives, but also reduces the physical and financial burden of cancer care. However, early detection and prevention are severely underfunded and undervalued. Given the inefficacy of treating advanced-stage cancers, it is vital to shift our focus to proactive, preventive care for asymptomatic high-risk individuals.

As I propose in a three-tier anti-cancer strategy, proactive systemic early cancer detection and intervention should be the top priority. Rationally, allocating more than half of all cancer care resources to early detection and prevention strategies is necessary, serving as the effective defense against cancer.

Transitioning from our current reactive sick care system to a proactive, preventive healthcare model on a societal level poses numerous challenges. The entrenched interests within this intricate healthcare ecosystem, which consumes 17.8% of the US GDP (USD 4.15 trillion in 2021)—exceeding the GDPs of Germany (USD 3.9 trillion) and India (USD 3.0 trillion)—will be a major hurdle. Due to the deeply vested financial interests across various segments, redirecting healthcare resources towards early detection and prevention will be unsettling for many elements of the current costly and inefficient "sick care" system, likely encountering strong resistance and intense criticism.

Achieving a paradigm shift toward early detection and preventive care requires the collective effort and collaboration of diverse stakeholders. This includes individuals, healthcare providers, corporations, foundations, societies, insurance

Three Tiers of Anti-Cancer Strategies:

Tier 1: Proactive Systemic Early Cancer Detection and Intervention

Catching precancerous and cancerous lesions at early, curable stages for early intervention using emerging systemic cancer screening tests (whole-body MRI and blood ctDNA tests) in addition to current single-site screening tests.

Tier 2: Cancer Prevention by Mitigating Modifiable Risk Factors

Preventing or inhibiting cancer development by following current guidelines to reduce various modifiable risk factors.

Tier 3: Reactive, Symptom-Triggered Diagnosis and Treatment

A full array of treatment options will be used for a fraction of patients who are diagnosed with advanced-stage cancers despite early detection and prevention efforts as a last resort.

companies, and government agencies. Each must contribute to transitioning toward a healthcare model focused on prevention and early detection. Future initiatives should prioritize expanding imaging and diagnostic centers, as well as outpatient surgery facilities for early intervention. This shift will reduce the reliance on comprehensive cancer centers and hospital care for advanced cancer patients, ultimately saving lives and lowering healthcare costs and burdens.

Public awareness about the importance of cancer screening and early detection is critical. Given the challenges in increasing or reallocating government funding for these purposes, overcoming the numerous obstacles to this fundamental shift will take considerable time. Visionary and passionate advocates like Mary Lasker are essential in championing the advancement and efficient adoption of innovative cancer screening and early detection technologies.

Internal Self-Portraits with Whole-Body MRI for Preventive Care

The journey from the first self-portrait photograph to the advent of MRI and its evolution into a tool for preventive healthcare through whole-body MRI scans represents a transformative narrative. This pioneering use of MRI technology unveils the intricate workings of the human body, redefining how we perceive and safeguard our well-being.

The narrative begins in 1839, with Robert Cornelius, an American photography pioneer, etching his name into history by capturing what is believed to be the first photographic self-portrait. This moment transcends mere artistic expression and symbolizes the birth of humanity's ability to document and study the self through visual means. Cornelius' innovation laid the foundational principles of photographic technology, influencing various fields, including the emerging medical imaging domain.

As the story progresses, the late 19th and early 20th centuries mark the advent of medical imaging, catalyzed by Wilhelm Conrad Roentgen's groundbreaking discovery of X-rays in 1895. This revolutionary technology ushered in a new era, allowing physicians to peer inside the human body without surgery. Subsequent advancements, such as the introduction of CT scans in the 1970s, further expanded the horizons of internal imaging.

However, the introduction of MRI in 1977 by Raymond Damadian and his colleagues indeed marked a paradigm shift. Unlike its predecessors, which relied on ionizing radiation, MRI utilized the harmless interplay of magnetic fields and radio waves to produce exquisitely detailed images of the body's internal structures. This safe and innovative approach provided unparalleled clarity in visualizing soft tissues and paved the way for more frequent diagnostic use, heralding a new era of medical exploration.

In a crescendo of technological advancement, MRI technology evolved to enable comprehensive whole-body scans, representing a leap in preventive healthcare. These scans, akin to a "full-body portrait" of an individual's internal health, unveil invaluable insights once shrouded in mystery. My whole-body MRI image, generated by Prenuvo in 2022 after a 60-minute scan, stands as a testament to the transformative power of this technology in preventive care.

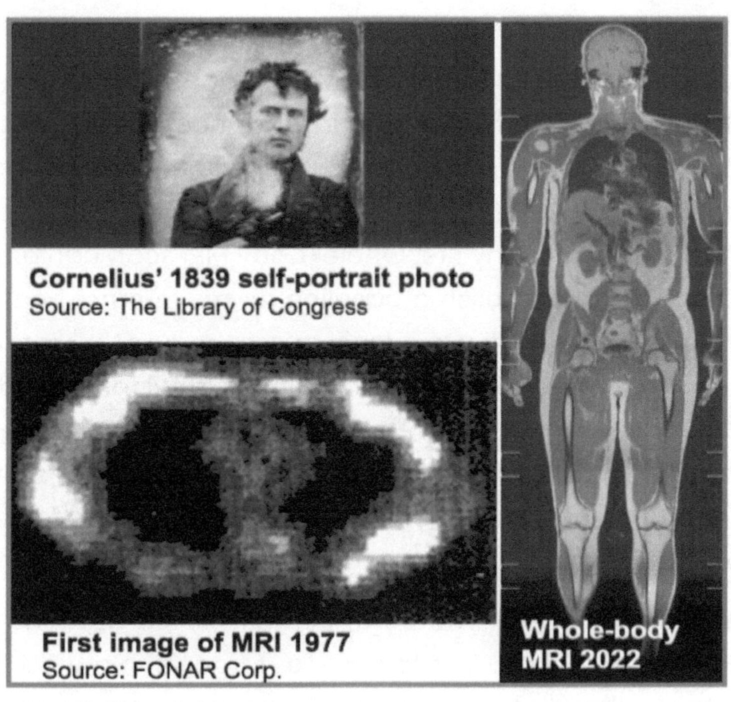

The First Whole-Body MRI Scan:

A Baseline for Personalized Preventive Care

As the Roman poet Virgil aptly coined the idiom 2,000 years ago, "The greatest wealth is health.". Indeed, it behooves us to strive earnestly to maintain our health and wellbeing for as long as possible.

The human body is an intricate enigma, and we still lack comprehensive understanding of our individual internal processes. While blood biomarker tests provide critical insights into organ health, they often fail to detect early-stage diseases since organs can compensate for significant functional loss. Highly sensitive whole-body MRI scans can shed light on this "black box" by revealing early signs of disease. People tend to respond more strongly to visual images like MRI scans than to numerical data from blood tests, making them more likely to take preventive actions when they can see pathological changes visually.

Many chronic diseases begin at a young age, progressing slowly and silently. This underscores the importance of early detection. Spotting disease signs early enables lifestyle changes or medical interventions that can significantly alter the disease's course. I wish I had undergone my first whole-body MRI scan earlier, ideally around age 30, to establish a baseline for my internal health. This initial scan is crucial as it provides a reference point for monitoring changes over time. Longitudinal imaging is ideal for early disease detection, allowing for the tracking of subtle changes and abnormalities throughout the body and offering opportunities for early intervention and personalized preventive care for various medical conditions as a person ages.

Understanding the importance of establishing a baseline with a whole-body MRI scan, I decided to forgo a planned trip to celebrate my daughter's upcoming 25th birthday. Instead, I chose to allocate the travel funds to gift her a whole-body MRI. Although she is currently young and healthy, I believe this is the best gift for her future well-being, providing a valuable reference for personalized preventive care. If she's anxious about potential findings, she need not review the scan report herself; I can examine it and inform her only if there are issues needing attention. This way, she can simply store the valuable image data for future use in her personalized preventive care.

Beyond Cancer: Early Detection of Other Medical Conditions

Whole-body MRI scans possess a remarkable capacity to detect early signs of disease across all body parts simultaneously, from brain tumors and arterial anomalies to musculoskeletal disorders. The manifold benefits include:

- Early Disease Detection: Many severe diseases, including cancers, neurological disorders, and vascular conditions, often remain undetected until they reach advanced and potentially life-threatening stages. A baseline whole-body MRI scan can reveal these conditions in their earliest phases, significantly improving the chances of successful treatment and recovery.

- Longitudinal Health Monitoring: By establishing a comprehensive health baseline, individuals and their healthcare providers can monitor changes over time, identifying subtle shifts that may signal disease onset. This longitudinal approach proves invaluable in managing age-related conditions and preempting their progression.

- Personalized Health Insights: A whole-body MRI offers an all-encompassing overview of an individual's health status, providing insights that can be used to tailor personal health strategies. This may manifest in dietary adjustments, exercise regimens, or preventive medicine meticulously designed to address the specific health risks identified during the scan. This inclusivity of whole-body MRI enables the detection of unexpected health issues that more targeted screening protocols might overlook.

While cancer detection remains a primary focus, whole-body MRI is equally invaluable for diagnosing a wide array of other diseases. Cardiovascular conditions, such as aneurysms, can be identified through detailed imaging of blood vessels and the heart. Early detection of these issues allows for proactive management, significantly reducing the risk of severe complications like heart attacks and strokes.

Whole-body MRI is also pivotal in identifying neurological disorders, including multiple sclerosis, brain tumors, and spinal cord abnormalities. Its capability to capture high-resolution images of the brain and spinal cord facilitates the early detection and treatment of these potentially debilitating conditions. Additionally, musculoskeletal disorders, such as arthritis, osteoporosis, and soft tissue injuries, can be effectively diagnosed with whole-body MRI, enabling early intervention and improved patient outcomes.

Moreover, whole-body MRI offers a comprehensive view of the body, allowing for the simultaneous assessment of multiple organ systems. This holistic approach is particularly beneficial in diagnosing systemic diseases that may affect various parts of the body. The detailed images produced by MRI can reveal subtle changes in tissues and organs, aiding in the early diagnosis of diseases that might not yet present symptoms.

Case Study: Unraveling the Enigma of Intracranial Aneurysms. In a recent study led by Prenuvo, the prevalence of intracranial aneurysms (IAs) in North America was meticulously investigated by analyzing whole-body MRI scans, alongside exploring lifestyle and medical risk factors. With a sample size of 23,352 participants—51% males and 49% females, with an average age of 51.6 years—this study illuminates the intricate interplay between modifiable factors and the formation of these potentially life-threatening vascular anomalies. The findings are both enlightening and sobering: a total of 484 (2%) IAs were detected, with a higher prevalence among females (2.2%) compared to males (1.7%). While most IAs were small, with only 7 (4%) larger than 7mm, the study underscores the critical roles of age, hypertension, family history, and cardiovascular health in developing these insidious lesions.

Whole-body MRI has a wide range of applications in preventive healthcare. For example, Dr. Attariwala and his team studied MRI images of 10,125 healthy individuals and discovered that exercise-related physical activity is linked to increased brain volumes, suggesting potential neuroprotective effects. They also found that higher levels of subcutaneous fat are associated with brain volume loss.

Prenuvo is believed to have the world's largest normative dataset for whole-body imaging. This extensive collection enables their AI researchers to collaborate with leading academics to define what constitutes "normal" aging. Such insights are vital because traditional healthcare has emphasized disease treatment over health assessment. Evaluating "normal" based on factors such as age, gender, and ethnicity offers valuable context. They are developing AI models to enhance the precision and quantitativeness of imaging. Through regular MRI scans, AI facilitates the creation of a comprehensive longitudinal view of how each body part ages, allowing for the establishment of a personalized baseline. Many of their groundbreaking findings in preventive care by Prenuvo have been shared with the healthcare and scientific communities through numerous published papers and abstracts, as well as conference presentations.

As modern preventive healthcare continues to evolve, the integration of advanced imaging techniques like MRI transforms the early detection of diseases in asymptomatic, healthy individuals.

Early Detection Initiatives in Leading Medical Centers

Dana-Farber's Centers for Early Detection and Interception

At the forefront of the revolution in cancer care, Dana-Farber Cancer Institute has established the Center for Early Detection and Interception (CEDI), underscoring its commitment to eradicating cancer. This innovative initiative represents a forward-thinking approach, emphasizing the critical importance of identifying and treating cancer at its earliest stages.

Dana-Farber's CEDI aims to revolutionize cancer diagnosis and treatment by prioritizing early detection and interception. Through this ambitious endeavor, the institute seeks to enhance patient outcomes, reduce treatment-related costs, and ultimately lower cancer mortality rates by catching the disease early—a mission that resonates deeply with cancer patients. The CEDI employs a multidisciplinary approach, integrating advanced technologies and cutting-edge research methodologies.

Center for Cancer Prevention and Early Detection at City of Hope

City of Hope's Center for Cancer Prevention and Early Detection is dedicated to advancing new technologies in cancer risk prediction, early detection, and monitoring. The center's goals are to prevent or detect cancer at its earliest stages and implement methods that reach diverse, rural, and underserved populations. By uniting researchers from various academic disciplines, the center translates findings on cancer prevention, early detection, and monitoring into clinical practice. The focus is on developing key research findings and novel technologies, such as non-invasive blood tests and imaging, which have the potential to detect cancers years before conventional diagnostic methods.

Many leading medical centers in the United States, including **Johns Hopkins** and **MD Anderson**, are shifting the paradigm in cancer care by establishing Centers for Cancer Prevention and Early Detection. These centers integrate cutting-edge research with practical preventive healthcare services. This innovative approach focuses on stopping cancer before it starts or catching it at its earliest stages, fundamentally transforming patient outcomes. By promoting early detection through advanced screening technologies like liquid biopsies and enhanced imaging techniques, these centers are setting new standards in preventive cancer care.

Transforming Early Detection: Integrating AI into Whole-Body MRI and ctDNA Tests

Early detection and prevention have always been pivotal in modern healthcare. Recent advancements in AI, medical imaging, and liquid biopsy technologies are revolutionizing this space. Integrating state-of-the-art techniques like whole-body MRI, ctDNA tests, and AI-driven decision support systems promises to redefine how we detect cancer and other diseases early, heralding a new era in preventive care.

Whole-body MRI has proven itself to be a robust tool for comprehensive anatomical screening, capable of identifying abnormalities throughout the body in one non-invasive examination. It has already shown efficacy in cancer screening for genetically predisposed individuals, and its broader potential in preventive care is actively being explored. Complementing this anatomical insight, liquid biopsy techniques such as ctDNA analysis offer a glimpse into the molecular landscape of diseases. By detecting and analyzing circulating tumor DNA fragments in the bloodstream, these tests can potentially identify cancer or other conditions at an early stage, even before they manifest on imaging.

While individually powerful, whole-body MRI and ctDNA analysis reach their full potential when combined with AI. AI algorithms, trained on extensive datasets of medical images, genomic data, and clinical information, can discern intricate patterns and signatures associated with various diseases.

The fusion of anatomical data from whole-body MRI with molecular insights from ctDNA analysis, processed through AI models, unlocks unparalleled diagnostic precision. AI can identify subtle abnormalities that human observers might overlook and integrate diverse data streams to offer comprehensive risk assessments and personalized screening recommendations.

Integrating these technologies, however, presents several challenges. Standardizing imaging protocols, data acquisition, and interpretation guidelines is crucial for ensuring consistent and reliable results across different healthcare facilities. Critical considerations include managing incidental findings, evaluating cost-effectiveness, and providing patient acceptance and compliance. Furthermore, the ethical implications of comprehensive screening approaches must be meticulously addressed. Issues regarding data privacy, informed consent, and the potential for overdiagnosis and overtreatment require careful navigation. Collaboration among healthcare professionals, researchers, policymakers, and ethicists is essential to establish robust ethical frameworks and guidelines, safeguarding patient well-being while maximizing the benefits of these transformative technologies.

In summary, the convergence of AI, whole-body MRI, and ctDNA tests marks a monumental leap in early detection and preventive care. AI-powered systemic early detection across the entire body offers the most effective and practical approach to defeating cancer by identifying most cancers at their early, curable stages. These systemic early detection tests should be adopted promptly to save lives.

Individual-Driven Systemic Early Detection

"The greatest wealth is health."
Virgil
"Spotting cancer at an early stage saves lives."
Cancer Research UK

The drive of this book centers on a pivotal inquiry:

How can we take action now to effectively minimize the risk of succumbing to cancer?

After a thorough assessment of the landscape of cancer care detailed in the earlier chapters, I have distilled several key insights:

- Late-stage cancer remains largely incurable despite advancements in targeted therapy and immunotherapy. Moreover, a cure for metastatic cancer is not even on the horizon.

- Aging is the biggest risk factor for cancer, obstructing efficacious prevention even for those who lead healthy lifestyles and minimize all modifiable risk factors.

- Early detection stands as the most effective and feasible strategy for defeating cancer.

- Unfortunately, there are significant gaps in current cancer screening tests, which are limited to just a few cancer types. The majority of all cancer deaths result from cancers, such as pancreatic, ovarian, liver, kidney, stomach, esophageal, bone, and brain cancers, without existing screening tests.

In this final chapter, I will share a practical plan to fill the significant gaps in current cancer screenings to minimize cancer risk. This proactive plan for systemic early detection, aimed at catching most cancers at early, curable stages, should be applicable to all individuals over the age of 50, regardless of their health status or family history.

Early Detection Saves Lives

The cumulative data had spoken, and its message was clear: early detection of cancer significantly boosts survival rates, while advanced cancers remained largely incurable.

Data stand true in front of us, illustrating this fact.

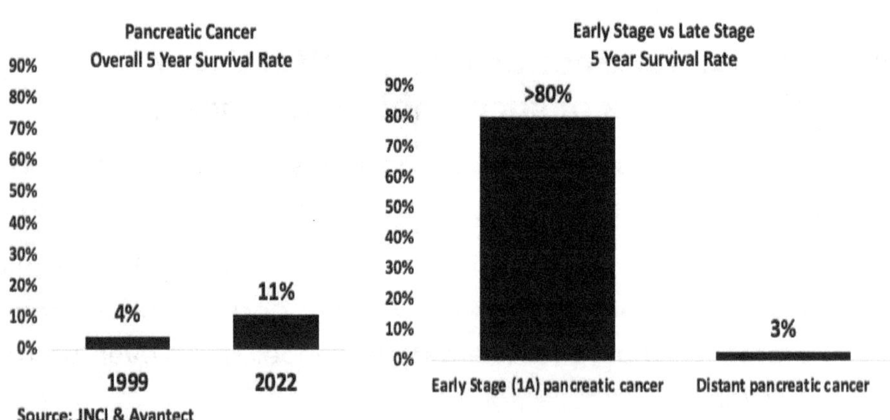

For example, significant progress has been made in treating pancreatic cancer. As illustrated in the accompanying figure, the five-year overall survival rate for pancreatic cancer had risen impressively from 4% in 1999 to 11% in 2022, an impressive increase of 175%, which is duly celebrated. However, the survival rates between early and late-stage pancreatic cancer were starkly different: over 80% for early-stage compared to just 3% for late-stage. In 2023, about 64,050 new cases of pancreatic cancer were diagnosed in the U.S., with 50,550 deaths, surpassing the approximately 40,000 car accident deaths per year.

This highlighted that despite advancements in treatment, the improvement in survival rates for patients with late-stage pancreatic cancer remained dismal.

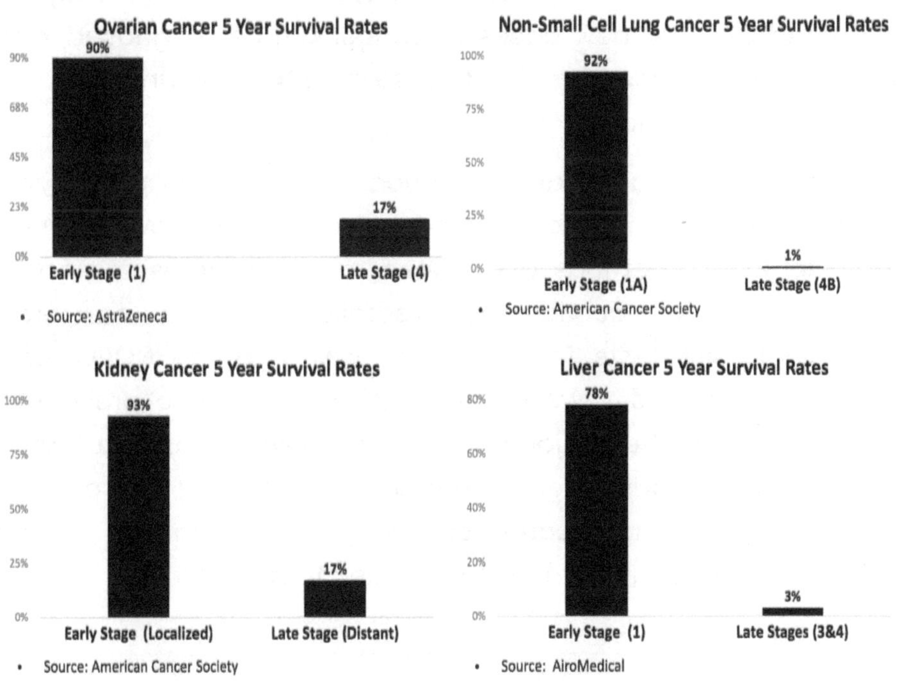

Survival data consistently highlights a stark contrast between late-stage and early-stage cancer outcomes. Patients diagnosed with early-stage cancers such as ovarian, lung, kidney, and liver cancer, have a much higher survival rate.

This underscores the vital role of early detection as the most effective strategy for conquering cancer. Hence, shifting our focus and resources from treatment to early detection is imperative, aiming to catch cancer in its early, curable stages.

Huge Gaps in Cancer Prevention and Early Detection

Prevention should be the primary strategy to combat cancer, stopping cancer development from its inception. Despite some success in cancer prevention measures, such as smoking cessation, vaccinations against cancer-causing viruses (HPV and HBV), and reducing environmental exposure to carcinogens, cancer incidence continues to rise both in the US and globally. An estimated 2,001,140 new cases of cancer will be diagnosed, and 611,720 people will die from the disease in 2024 in the United States (NCI Cancer Statistics).

Cancer screening and early detection, as secondary prevention, aim to detect cancer before symptoms emerge. However, current early detection methods are limited to a few types of cancer —namely breast, cervical, colorectal, and lung cancers— using single-site tests for each. According to the NORC, only 14% of cancer cases were detected through these preventive screening tests. The majority of cancer deaths were attributed to cancers without recommended screening protocols. This reality underscores critical gaps in current cancer prevention and early detection that need to be rectified.

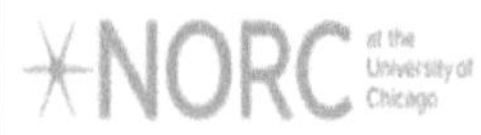

Major Cancer Types without Recommended Screening Tests
Pancreatic Cancer
Ovarian Cancer
Stomach (Gastric) Cancer
Liver Cancer
Kidney (Renal) Cancer
Brain Cancer
Esophageal Cancer
Gallbladder Cancer
Small Intestine Cancer
Bladder Cancer
Lung Cancer (Non-Smokers)

Case Study: Colonoscopy Still the Sole Recommended Cancer Screening for Non-Smoking Men

Imagine a world where the flip of a coin determines your fate. For a non-smoking male like me, this isn't far from reality. We face a 40-50% chance of hearing the dreaded words, "You have cancer," at some point in our lives. Yet, despite these daunting odds, our defenses seem woefully inadequate.

The US Preventive Services Task Force, our nation's guardian of screening recommendations, offers us a single, local shield for colorectal cancer: the colonoscopy. This lone sentinel guards our colorectal health, leaving the rest of our body in vast, defenseless territory.

Cancer Screening Tests Currently Recommended by USPSTF for Non-Smoking Men

Cancer Type	Screening Test	Population	Frequency
Colorectal Cancer	Colonoscopy, Sigmoidoscopy, FIT, FOBT	Adults aged 45 to 75	Varies by test (1–10 years)
Prostate Cancer	Prostate-Specific Antigen (PSA) Test	Men aged 55 to 69	Individual decision

The story of the colonoscopy is one of perseverance and prolonged adoption. Picture two pioneering doctors, William Wolff and Hiromi Shinya, huddled over their creation in a New York City hospital in 1969. Their invention, capable of peering into the furthest reaches of the colon, was revolutionary. By 1973, they had demonstrated its potential to intercept cancer's foot soldiers—polyps—before they could establish their deadly reign.

Yet, like many significant innovations, the colonoscopy's journey to widespread acceptance was a marathon. It wasn't until the 1990s that it began to receive its due recognition. The year 1997 marked a turning point, as the National Polyp Study conclusively proved what Wolff and Shinya had known all along: removing these precancerous polyps significantly reduced the incidence of colorectal cancer.

But what of the rest of our bodies? For non-smoking men, the colonoscopy stands alone, besides the optional PSA test. There are no recommended screenings for the myriads of other cancers that may be silently growing within us as we age. It's a sobering thought—that we must wait for symptoms to appear before seeking help. By this time, the enemy may have already spread and fortified its position, becoming nearly undefeatable.

The guidelines governing our cancer screening protocols are crafted with the best intentions. They aim to strike a delicate balance between benefit and risk, cost and effectiveness, on a societal scale. But in this grand equation, individual lives become mere data points. If you're unlucky enough to develop a cancer for which no screening is recommended, and it's caught too late, it's dismissed as a simple misfortune.

Yet, I find myself unwilling to accept this status quo. In a world where technology advances at a breakneck pace, it seems almost inconceivable that we still rely solely on a technique developed over half a century ago. This realization begs the question: What other promising cancer screening technologies have emerged since 1969? In this age of unprecedented scientific progress, new sentinels are likely ready to join the colonoscopy in its vigilant watch over our health.

As we stand on the precipice of a new era in medical technology, it's time to look beyond the limitations of current guidelines. It's time to explore the cutting edge of cancer detection and seek out emerging technologies that could tip the odds in our favor. In this high-stake game of life and death, we need every advantage we can get.

Technology Breakthroughs in Systemic Early Detection

New hope has emerged in the field where warriors battle the dreaded cancer. Recent breakthrough technologies, including whole-body MRI scans and blood ctDNA tests, have made the once-impossible dream of systemic early detection across the entire body with a single test a reality. The sensitivity and specificity of these tests have been validated through clinical trials and use. Moreover, the increasing integration of AI with medical imaging and diagnosis is revolutionizing the field. The convergence of AI, detection technologies, and large data makes these innovative systemic early detection tests more effective, convenient, and accessible. The early detection of cancer and precancer lesions by integrating systemic early detection and AI is where our brightest future resides.

Aging: The Biggest, yet Non-modifiable, Risk Factor

A somber reality is that no one can escape the threat of cancer, even if you make great efforts and do everything perfectly to prevent it by diligently following guidelines and eliminating all modifiable cancer risk factors. For example, at the age of 55, you exercise regularly, eat a healthy diet, maintain a normal body weight, do not smoke or drink, and have no HBV and HPV infection and no family history of cancer. While these factors certainly reduce your risk of cancer, you are still at high risk solely because of your age.

According to the National Cancer Institute, approximately 40.5% of men and women will be diagnosed with cancer at some point during their lifetimes. While cancer can affect individuals of any age, including the young, the incidence of cancer significantly increases after the age of 40. In the US, the median age at cancer diagnosis is 66. Recent research shows accelerated aging linked to increased cancer risk in younger adults. Aging stands as the biggest risk factor for cancer, making efficacious prevention unachievable, even with optimal management of all modifiable risk factors, including healthy lifestyles and vaccinations. The reasons for aging in cancer are multi-faceted, such as the accumulation of induced and random mutations, aging immunity, and aging-associated inflammation, as discussed earlier.

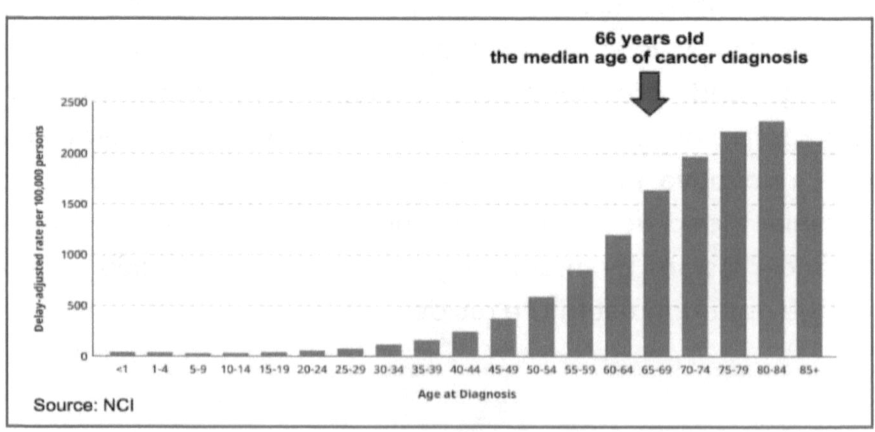

Therefore, anyone over the age of 40, especially those 50 or older, is at high risk of cancer, regardless of their family history, overall health and socioeconomic status, and efforts to reduce modifiable risk factors.

No Choice, But Proactive Early Detection

Here is a summary of the current status of cancer care as detailed in previous chapters:

Current Status of Cancer Care

- **Aging is the biggest, yet non-modifiable, risk factor, thus hindering prevention and increasing cancer incidence.**

- **Current recommended cancer screening tests are only for colorectal cancer and lung cancer (for smokers) for both men and women, plus breast and cervical cancer for women.**

- **Symptomatic, late-stage cancer remains largely incurable despite recent advances in targeted therapy and immunotherapy.**

- **The decline in US cancer mortality rate is primarily due to cancer prevention and early detection.**

A critical evaluation of cancer treatment, prevention, and screening/early detection reveals that regular, systemic early detection across the entire body is the most effective and feasible strategy to defeat cancer. Hence, it is crucial to actively explore and adopt innovative technologies for early cancer detection.

The cancer miracle that will emerge is not a cure for advanced cancer; it is the systemic early detection across the whole body to catch most cancers at their early, curable stages!

Missing Opportunities for Early Detection

The ancient tale of the Sword of Damocles vividly captures the essence of living under the threat of cancer—a word that strikes fear into many hearts. Just the mention of cancer can conjure images of suffering, loss, and an uncertain future. This fear is so overwhelming that numerous individuals go to great lengths to avoid facing the risk altogether. Often driven by a profound sense of fear and powerlessness, the prospect of confronting cancer can seem terrifying. Fear is a natural human response to the unknown. Cancer, with its myriad forms and unpredictable course, represents one of the most formidable unknowns in modern life.

Avoiding cancer screenings due to the fear of unknown findings is a significant issue with serious health consequences. Many individuals forgo screenings because they are afraid of discovering a potentially life-threatening condition. This fear of the unknown can paralyze, leading to procrastination or complete avoidance. Without screenings, cancer can progress silently to advanced, metastatic stages, which are largely incurable. Thus, the avoidance of cancer screening results in missed opportunities to catch cancer early when it is often curable. "A huge body of evidence shows that cancer isn't what kills us. It is cancer caught at later stages that kills people," wrote Dr. Cristian Tomasetti, director of the Center for Prevention and Early Detection at City of Hope.

Action Plan: Becoming a Prudent Adopter of Systemic Early Detection

I posed a solemn question to myself: If I were diagnosed with advanced pancreatic or liver cancer, despite following recommended prevention and screening guidelines, and succumbed to it even after receiving the best available treatments, who would be to blame?

The answer is stark: No one; it is merely a twist of fate—my own bad luck.

This prompted a subsequent question: What action could I take to minimize the risk of succumbing to cancer beyond current deficient screening guidelines?

To me, the answer is clear: systemic early detection throughout the entire body to catch most cancer types at their early, curable stages.

This raises a further question: When should I adopt these emerging systemic early-detection tests to fill the vast gaps in current cancer screening?

The dilemma of whether to act or wait always preoccupies my mind when considering the timing of adopting new systemic early detection tests.

Solely because of my age of over 50, I am an asymptomatic healthy individual at a high risk of cancer. I am resolute in making every effort to minimize the risk of dying from cancer. Whole-body MRI and ctDNA tests are now at the forefront of systemic cancer screening. However, the regulatory approval process for new screening tests, particularly for whole-body MRI, is a lengthy and complex journey that may well take several decades. For someone at high risk like me, waiting that long is not a good option.

To fill the huge gaps in existing cancer screening tests, I've embraced these systemic early detection tests, becoming an early adopter to minimize the risk of dying from cancer.

In the text box, I outline my approach to minimizing cancer risk. I undergo an annual whole-body MRI scan and a blood ctDNA test (Galleri MCED test), complemented with imaging and biomarker detection technologies spaced six months apart. This schedule maximizes the likelihood of detecting cancer at its earliest stages.

Whole-body MRI provides visual evidence of potential tumors or abnormalities, while a ctDNA test detect molecular signals from cancer cells. This synergistic method not only enhances sensitivity and accuracy but also aims to catch cancer at its earliest, most curable stages. Certainly, the frequency of taking these systemic screening tests can be adjusted based on the test findings and cost concerns, ranging from annually to every several years.

Proactive Early Cancer Detection for Asymptomatic High-Risk Individuals:

- **Whole-body MRI scan and blood ctDNA test, with complementary detection technologies, for systemic early cancer detection cross the whole body annually or regularly.**

- **Single-site cancer screening for five types of cancers, including colonoscopy, low-dose chest CT scans, mammograms, HPV-Pap smear tests, and PSA tests, adhering to current guidelines.**

It's important to note that these new systemic early detection tests complement, rather than replace, current single-site cancer screenings. I continue to adhere to existing cancer screening guidelines, such as colonoscopy. Although I am a non-smoker and do not qualify for a chest CT scan under current guidelines, I choose to undergo these scans every few years without insurance coverage due to the rising incidence of lung cancer in non-smokers. Additionally, I have an annual PSA test, as I find this biomarker data valuable. Furthermore, I make efforts to prevent cancer by reducing modifiable risk factors as much as possible.

In summary, the proactive, systemic early detection approach I've adopted represents the best current option for minimizing cancer mortality by detecting most cancers at their early, curable stages. This strategy could be applicable to other high-risk individuals in their fight against cancer.

User-Friendly Deployment of Systemic Early Detection Tests

Both systemic early detection tests are convenient, require minimal pre-test preparation, and cause minimal discomfort. I typically schedule the whole-body MRI during a lunch break, and the ctDNA blood draw at a clinical diagnostic lab in the morning on my way to work. Unlike invasive single-site tests like colonoscopies—which require unpleasant pre-test preparation, sedation during the procedure, and someone to drive you home afterward—these new systemic cancer detection tests are remarkably easy to undertake.

Personally, I find the colonoscopy procedure intimidating, but I almost look forward to the annual whole-body MRI. This scan allows me to track internal changes and monitor my overall wellbeing, all with minimal discomfort.

Integrating AI into Systemic Early Detection: Maximizing Early Detection While Minimizing Harm

The "do no harm" principle, known in Latin as "primum non nocere," is a cornerstone of medical ethics, originating from the Hippocratic Oath taken by ancient Greek physicians. This principle underscores the necessity of carefully balancing the benefits of a treatment or procedure against its risks and potential for harm.

The Pitfalls of Systemic Early Cancer Detection:

- **False Positives or Negatives:**
  - **Unnecessary follow-up examinations**
  - **False sense of security with potentially undetected tumors**
- **Overdiagnosis and Overtreatment: Particularly prevalent in prostate cancer and thyroid cancer**
- **Mental Stress**
- **Cost**

Earlier, chapters 6-9 delve into the pitfalls of these systemic early detection tests, emphasizing the critical need to address these issues to avoid causing more harm than good. Detailed strategies for mitigating these pitfalls, drawing from my personal experience and knowledge of these technologies, are deliberated in earlier chapters.

Until recently, systemic cancer screening tests capable of detecting multiple cancer types throughout the body with a single test were unavailable. Both healthcare providers and patients are still familiarizing themselves with these screenings, which are in the nascent stages of adoption. Major obstacles to widespread implementation include high costs, the need for extensive training, and the lack of established guidelines for routine use. Additionally, regulatory challenges present further hurdles, and concerns about false positives, overdiagnosis, and the psychological effects of incidental findings persist.

AI is swiftly revolutionizing numerous fields, and medical diagnostics is no exception. While AI's impact on medical diagnostics has been limited until now, recent breakthroughs are reshaping the landscape. By integrating AI with systemic early detection methods, the sensitivity and specificity of diagnostic tests are significantly enhanced, resulting in fewer false positives and negatives. AI integration accelerates automation, reduces costs, and enhances accessibility. In essence, the incorporation of AI is improving the accuracy, efficiency, and accessibility of whole-body MRI and ctDNA tests, positioning these technologies at the forefront of early cancer detection.

In essence, the pitfalls of these systemic early detection tests, such as whole-body MRI and ctDNA tests, can be overcome with concerted efforts. These AI-powered detection tests have the potential to identify most cancers at their early, curable stages effectively.

Individual-Driven Systemic Early Detection: Taking Action

The current central component in combating cancer is reactive, ineffective symptom-driven diagnosis and the treatment of often advanced, incurable cancers. Moreover, current cancer prevention and single-site screening measures have proven ineffective in general, as evidenced by the continuing rise in total cancer incidence and mortality both in the US and globally. A thorough evaluation of advances in cancer treatment, prevention, and early detection indicates that systemic early detection is the most effective way to defeat cancer.

Technological advancements, particularly in whole-body MRI, ctDNA tests, and AI, have transformed the fight against cancer by making systemic early detection across the whole body to catch most cancers at early, curable stages a reality.

Early detection undeniably saves lives. Whole-body MRI and ctDNA tests have demonstrated their ability to detect early-stage cancers. However, the debate over the benefits and drawbacks of preventive whole-body MRI and ctDNA tests is likely to persist for decades, as definitive evidence of reducing cancer mortality from randomized controlled trials in asymptomatic populations may not be available in the foreseeable future.

At a societal level, the recommendation and adoption of these emerging systemic early detection tests will take a long time due to various requirements and obstacles. Medical professionals are constrained by medical and health insurance guidelines, leading to their cautious attitude and approach toward adopting emerging life-saving technologies.

The dire reality is this: no one can save you if diagnosed with advanced cancer, such as pancreatic or liver cancer, at a late stage, even with unlimited resources at your disposal.

Individuals at high risk of cancer, like me, should take proactive steps to minimize the risk of succumbing to it by going beyond the current inadequate screening and prevention guidelines. Systemic early detection throughout the entire body is the most effective and practical way to defeat cancer, as detailed earlier. While early adoption of systemic cancer screenings is not forthright or inexpensive, at a personal level, we have the power to take our own initiative by adopting emerging systemic early detection tests, armed with knowledge, effort and determination to beat cancer.

As we reach the end of our grand tour through the battlefield against cancer, I hope we all come to the same conclusion:

The key to defeating cancer lies not in finding a cure for late-stage cancer, but in systemic early detection, empowered by AI integration.

By understanding the potential and limitations of these detection technologies, you are equipped to make informed, science-based decisions about when and how to adopt these innovative tests to catch most cancers early in consultation with healthcare providers.

Let's Take Action to Catch Most Cancers Early Through Revolutionary AI-Powered Systemic Detection!

ENDNOTE--REVIEW REQUEST

If you enjoy reading this book and agree with the pressing need to shift from ineffective and costly sick care to preventive early detection and health care, please consider leaving a review on Amazon and other book sites.

Your review not only helps new readers find this book but also amplifies the message of the vital importance of individual-driven, proactive early detection in defeating cancer.

Together, we can accelerate the transformative shift toward preventive health care and save our own lives and the lives of others.

GLOSSARY

Aging: The process of becoming older, a natural part of life that involves a gradual decline in physical and mental capacity.

AI (Artificial Intelligence): The simulation of human intelligence processes by machines, especially computer systems. These processes include learning, reasoning, and self-correction.

Antibody: A protein produced by the immune system that recognizes and binds to specific antigens to help fight infections and other foreign substances in the body.

Antibody-drug conjugate (ADC): A targeted cancer therapy that combines an antibody specific to cancer cells with a cytotoxic drug.

Biomarker: A biological molecule found in blood, other body fluids, or tissues that is a sign of a normal or abnormal process, or a condition or disease.

Bispecific antibody: An engineered antibody that binds to two different antigens or epitopes.

Bispecific T cell engager (BITE): A type of bispecific antibody that binds both to a T cell and a tumor cell, directing the immune system to attack the tumor.

Cancer: A disease characterized by the uncontrolled growth and metastasis of abnormal cells in the body.

Cancer screening: The process of checking for cancer in individuals who do not have symptoms of the disease.

Cancer early detection: The practice of using medical tests and procedures to detect cancer early in its development, often before symptoms appear.

CAR T cell therapy: Chimeric Antigen Receptor (CAR) T-cell therapy is a type of treatment in which a patient's T cells (a type of immune cell) are changed in the laboratory so they will attack cancer cells.

cfDNA (Cell-free DNA): DNA that is freely circulating in the bloodstream, originating from normal and tumor cells, used in clinical diagnostics.

Clinical Laboratory Improvement Amendments (CLIA): U.S. federal regulatory standards that apply to all clinical laboratory testing performed on humans.

ctDNA (Circulating tumor DNA): Tumor-derived fragmented DNA in the bloodstream that is not associated with cells. ctDNA can be used as a biomarker for cancer.

CT (Computed Tomography): An imaging procedure that uses special x-ray equipment to create detailed pictures, or scans, of areas inside the body.

Deep learning: A subset of machine learning involving neural networks with many layers that can learn from vast amounts of data.

DNA (Deoxyribonucleic Acid): The hereditary material in humans and almost all other organisms.

DNA methylation: A biochemical process involving the addition of a methyl group to the DNA molecule, often affecting gene expression.

False negatives: Test results that fail to detect a disease or condition when it is actually present.

False positives: Test results that wrongly indicate the presence of a disease or condition when it is not present.

Generative AI: A type of artificial intelligence that can generate new content, such as text, images, or music, often using deep learning models.

Graphics processing units (GPUs): Specialized electronic circuits designed to accelerate the processing of images and computations, particularly useful in AI and deep learning.

Immune checkpoint: A regulator of the immune system that, when activated, can diminish the immune response.

Immune checkpoint blockade: A form of cancer immunotherapy that uses antibodies to counteract checkpoints, thereby boosting the immune system's response against cancer cells.

Immunotherapy: Treatment that uses certain parts of a person's immune system to fight diseases such as cancer.

Indolent lesions: Slow-growing lesions that are unlikely to cause symptoms or death.

Indeterminate finding: A test result that is unclear and does not confirm whether a disease is present or absent.

Induced mutation: A genetic alteration caused by external factors such as radiation or chemicals.

Laboratory-Developed Tests (LDTs): Diagnostic tests developed and used within a single laboratory.

Large Language Models: Advanced AI systems that can understand and generate human-like text based on vast amounts of language data.

Liquid biopsy: A test done on a sample of blood to look for cancer cells or pieces of DNA from tumor cells.

Longitudinal imaging: Imaging tests performed over a period of time to track the progress of an abnormality or the effects of treatment.

Machine learning (ML): A branch of artificial intelligence that involves the creation of algorithms that can learn from and make predictions or decisions based on data.

MCED test (Multi-Cancer Early Detection test): A test designed to detect multiple types of cancer through biomarkers in the blood.

MRI (Magnetic Resonance Imaging): A non-invasive, non-radiation medical imaging technique used to create detailed images of the body's internal structures and physiological processes. MRI utilizes strong magnetic fields, radio waves, and field gradients to generate high-resolution images of organs, tissues, and the skeletal system.

MRI sequence: A specific setting or series of parameters used in an MRI exam to specifically highlight certain types of tissues and abnormalities.

MRI protocol: A predefined procedural strategy, based on the sequence settings, used to perform an MRI aimed at acquiring clinically relevant information.

Mutation: A change in the DNA sequence of a cell's genome, which can be caused by mistakes during DNA replication or by exposure to radiation or carcinogens.

NGS (Next Generation Sequencing): A method used to sequence DNA and RNA much more quickly and cheaply than older methods, facilitating genomic discoveries.

Oncogene: A gene that, when mutated or expressed at high levels, helps turn a normal cell into a tumor cell.

Over-diagnosis: The diagnosis of a disease or condition that will never cause symptoms or death during a patient's lifetime.

Over-treatment: The application of a medical treatment that is not necessary as it treats an overly diagnosed condition that would otherwise not cause harm.

Pixel: The smallest unit of a digital image, typically displayed on a digital display or represented in a digital image file.

Positive Predictive Value (PPV): A key metric in assessing the effectiveness of cancer screening tests. It measures the proportion of positive test results that are true positives, indicating the actual presence of cancer.

Random mutation: A mutation that occurs by chance and without any specific cause.

Scanxiety: Anxiety experienced by patients while taking scans or awaiting the results of medical scans.

Targeted therapy: A type of cancer treatment that uses drugs or other substances to precisely identify and attack cancer cells, usually while doing little damage to normal cells.

T cell: A type of lymphocyte (a subtype of white blood cell) that plays a central role in cell-mediated immunity.

Transformer Architecture: A neural network architecture that has been used to achieve significant advancements in natural language processing tasks.

The Tesla (T): The unit of magnetic flux density in the International System of Units (SI). Named after the inventor and electrical engineer Nikola Tesla, the unit measures the strength and intensity of magnetic fields. 1 Tesla = 1 Weber per square meter (Wb/m^2).

Tumor: An abnormal mass of tissue that results when cells divide more than they should or do not die when they should. Tumors can be benign or malignant with metastatic capacity.

Voxel: A volume pixel, representing a value on a regular grid in three-dimensional space, used in imaging analysis.

Whole-body MRI scan: An MRI scan of the whole body, instead of focusing on a particular organ or area of the body.

SELECTED BIBLIOGRAPHY

Chapter 1. Introduction: Still the Most Fearful Disease

- National Cancer Institute (NCI)- Cancer Moonshot. www.cancer.gov.
- National Cancer Institute. National Cancer Act of 1971.
- Lasker Foundation. Empress of All Maladies: Mary Lasker. https://laskerfoundation.org/empress-of-all-maladies-mary-lasker/
- Ferlay J, et al. Global Cancer Observatory: Cancer Today. Lyon: International Agency for Research on Cancer; 2020.
- Mukherjee S. The Emperor of All Maladies: A Biography of Cancer, 2010.
- Surh YJ. The 50-Year War on Cancer Revisited: Should We Continue to Fight the Enemy Within? J Cancer Prev. 26(4):219–223, 2021.
- The World Health Organization (WHO), Fact Sheets, Cancer. https://www.who.int/news-room/fact-sheets/detail/cancer

Chapter 2. The Enduring Challenge of Finding a Cure

- Bedard PL, et al. Small molecules, big impact: 20 years of targeted therapy in oncology. The Lancet. 395:1078-1088, 2020.
- Bonifant CL, et al. Toxicity and management in CAR T-cell therapy. Mol Ther Oncolytics. 3, 2016.
- Chen SY, Bagley J, Marasco WA. Intracellular antibodies as a new class of therapeutic molecules for gene therapy. Hum Gene Ther. 5:595-601, 1994.
- Daei Sorkhabi A, et al. The current landscape of CAR T-cell therapy for solid tumors: Mechanisms, research progress, challenges, and counterstrategies. Front Immunol. 14:1113882, 2023.

- Drago JZ, Modi S, Chandarlapaty S. Unlocking the potential of antibody–drug conjugates for cancer therapy. Nat Rev Clin Oncol. 18:327-344, 2021.
- Einsele H, et al. The BiTE (bispecific T-cell engager) platform: development and future potential of a targeted immuno-oncology therapy across tumor types. Cancer. 126:3192-3201, 2020.
- Goebeler ME, Bargou RC. T cell-engaging therapies—BiTEs and beyond. Nat Rev Clin Oncol. 17:418-434, 2020.
- June CH, et al. CAR T cell immunotherapy for human cancer. Science. 359:1361-1365, 2018.
- June CH, Sadelain M. Chimeric antigen receptor therapy. N Engl J Med. 379:64-73, 2018.
- Klein C, et al. The present and future of bispecific antibodies for cancer therapy. Nat Rev Drug Discov. 23:301-319, 2024.
- Krishnamurthy A, Jimeno A. Bispecific antibodies for cancer therapy: A review. Pharmacol Ther. 185:122-134, 2018.
- Lesch S, et al. Determinants of response and resistance to CAR T cell therapy. Semin Cancer Biol. 65, 2020.
- Maalej KM, et al. CAR-cell therapy in the era of solid tumor treatment: current challenges and emerging therapeutic advances. Mol Cancer. 22:20, 2023.
- Marasco WA, WA. Haseltine, and SY Chen. Design, intracellular expression, and activity of a human anti-human immunodeficiency virus type 1 gp120 single-chain antibody." Proceedings of the National Academy of Sciences 90:7889-7893, 1993
- Monberg TJ, et al. TIL therapy: facts and hopes. Clin Cancer Res. 29:3275-3283, 2023.
- Rafiq S, Hackett CS, Brentjens RJ. Engineering strategies to overcome the current roadblocks in CAR T cell therapy. Nat Rev Clin Oncol. 17:147-167, 2020.

- Rosenberg SA, Restifo NP. Adoptive cell transfer as personalized immunotherapy for human cancer. Science. 348:62-68, 2015.
- Sadelain M, Rivière I, Riddell S. Therapeutic T cell engineering. Nature. 545:423-431, 2017.
- Sanmamed MF, Chen L. A paradigm shift in cancer immunotherapy: from enhancement to normalization. Cell. 175:313-326, 2018.
- Seliger B, Massa C. Immune therapy resistance and immune escape of tumors. Cancers. 13:551, 2021.
- Sterner RC, Sterner RM. CAR-T cell therapy: current limitations and potential strategies. Blood Cancer J. 11:69, 2021.
- Topalian SL, et al. Neoadjuvant immune checkpoint blockade: A window of opportunity to advance cancer immunotherapy. Cancer Cell, 41:1551-1566, 2023.
- Vesely MD, Zhang T, Chen LP. Resistance mechanisms to anti-PD cancer immunotherapy. Annu Rev Immunol. 40:45-74, 2022.
- Wei PC, Duffy CR, Allison JP. Fundamental mechanisms of immune checkpoint blockade therapy. Cancer Discov. 8:1069-1086, 2018.
- Yang JC, Rosenberg SA. Adoptive T-cell therapy for cancer. Adv Immunol. 130:279-294, 2016.
- Ying Z, Huang XF, XX, Chen SY. A safe and potent anti-CD19 CAR T cell therapy. Nature Med. 25:947-953, 2019.
- Young RM, et al. Next-generation CAR T-cell therapies. Cancer Discov. 12:1625-1633, 2022.
- Zahavi D, Weiner L. Monoclonal antibodies in cancer therapy. Antibodies. 9:34, 2020.

Chapter 3. The Barrier of Non-modifiable Risk Factors in Prevention

- AACR Cancer Progress Report, 2023, Reducing the Risk of Cancer Development.

- Age and Cancer Risk. NCI. https://www.cancer.gov/about-cancer/causes-prevention/risk/age
- Age: the biggest cancer risk factor. Cancer Research UK. https://news.cancerresearchuk.org/2018/06/20/age-the-biggest-cancer-risk-factor
- Collatuzzo G, Boffetta P. Cancers Attributable to Modifiable Risk Factors: A Road Map for Prevention. Annu Rev Public Health. 44:279-300, 2023.
- Pasquale M, et al. Healthy Lifestyle and Cancer Risk: Modifiable Risk Factors to Prevent Cancer. Nutrients. 16:800, 2024.
- Mao JJ, et al. Integrative oncology: Addressing the global challenges of cancer prevention and treatment. CA Cancer J Clin. 72:144-164, 2022.
- NCI. Cancer Stat Facts: Cancer of Any Site. https://seer.cancer.gov/statfacts/html/all.html.
- Palshof FK, et al. Non-preventable cases of breast, prostate, lung, and colorectal cancer in 2050 in an elimination scenario of modifiable risk factors. Sci Rep. 14:8577, 2024.
- The World Health Organization. The International Agency for Research on Cancer (IARC). Global cancer burden growing, amidst mounting need for services, 2024.
- The World Health Organization. Preventing Cancer. https://www.who.int/activities/preventing-cancer.

Chapter 4. Huge Gaps in Early Detection

- American Cancer Society (ACS) Recommendations for Prostate Cancer Early Detection. https://www.cancer.org/cancer/types/prostate-cancer/detection-diagnosis-staging/acs-recommendations.html.
- Bratt O, et al. Screening for prostate cancer: Evidence, ongoing trials, policies and knowledge gaps. BMJ Oncol. 2:e000039, 2023.

- Bretthauer M, et al. Estimated lifetime gained with cancer screening tests: a meta-analysis of randomized clinical trials. JAMA Intern Med. 183:1196–1203, 2023.
- Carethers JM. Improving Noninvasive Colorectal Cancer Screening. N Engl J Med. 390:1045, 2024.
- CDC supports screening for breast, cervical, colorectal (colon), and lung cancers as recommended by the US Preventive Services Task Force (USPSTF).
- CDC. Cancer Screening Tests. https://www.cdc.gov/cancer/prevention/screening.html.
- Galeş LN, et al. Cancer Screening: Present Recommendations, the Development of Multi-Cancer Early Development Tests, and the Prospect of Universal Cancer Screening. Cancers. 16:1191, 2024.
- NCI. Screening Tests. https://www.cancer.gov/about-cancer/screening/screening-tests.
- Pastorino U, et al. Prolonged Lung Cancer Screening Reduced 10-year Mortality in the MILD Trial. Ann Oncol. 30:1162–1169, 2019.
- Philipson TJ, et al. The aggregate value of cancer screenings in the United States: full potential value and value considering adherence. BMC Health Serv Res. 23:829, 2023.
- Tomasetti C, Li L, Vogelstein B. Stem cell divisions, somatic mutations, cancer etiology, and cancer prevention. Science. 355:1330–1334, 2017.
- US Preventive Services Task US. Screening for cervical cancer: US preventive services task force recommendation statement. JAMA. 320:674–686, 2018.
- US Preventive Services Task Force. Final recommendation statement: breast cancer: screening. 2016.
- US Preventive Services Task Force. Final recommendation statement: prostate cancer. 2018.

- US Preventive Services Task Force. Screening for lung cancer: US preventive services task force recommendation statement. JAMA. 325:962-970, 2021.
- US Preventive Services Task Force. Screening for colorectal cancer: US Preventive Services Task Force recommendation statement. JAMA. 325:1965-1977, 2021.

Chapter 5. A New Path Forward—Systemic Early Detection

- American Cancer Society (ACS). Find Cancer Early. https://www.cancer.org/cancer/screening.html
- Cancer Research UK. Why is early cancer diagnosis important? https://www.cancerresearchuk.org/about-cancer/cancer-symptoms/why-is-early-diagnosis-important/1000
- Benford D, Bonar S. How City of Hope is leading the way in early cancer detection, prevention. 2024. https://www.cityofhope.org/early-cancer-detection-research.
- NCI. Prevention, Cancer Screening, and Early Diagnosis. https://healthcaredelivery.cancer.gov/prevention/
- NORC at the University of Chicago. Percent of Cancers Detected by Screening in the U.S. Available at https://cancerdetection.norc.org
- Ratner B, Bonislawski A. Early Detection: Catching Cancer When It's Curable. 2024.
- WHO. Promoting cancer early diagnosis. https://www.who.int/activities/promoting-cancer-early-diagnosis.

Chapter 6. Sensing the Tell-tale Signal of a Hidden Tumor

- Bai X, et al. PIK3CA and TP53 gene mutations in human breast cancer tumors frequently detected by ion torrent DNA sequencing. PLoS One. 9, 2014.

- Bruhm DC, et al. Single-molecule genome-wide mutation profiles of cell-free DNA for non-invasive detection of cancer. Nat Genet. 55:1301–1310, 2023.
- Chen KZ, et al. Circulating Tumor DNA Detection in Early-Stage Non-Small Cell Lung Cancer Patients by Targeted Sequencing. Sci Rep. 6:31985, 2016.
- Diehl F, et al. Detection and quantification of mutations in the plasma of patients with colorectal tumors. Proc Natl Acad Sci U S A. 102:16368-73, 2005.
- D'Arco N. Maximizing cancer early detection and minimizing harm. GRAIL. https://grail.com/stories/maximizing-cancer-early-detection-and-minimizing-harm, 2022.
- Fu X, Tao L, Zhang X. A chimeric virus-based probe unambiguously detects live circulating tumor cells with high specificity and sensitivity. Mol Ther Methods Clin Dev. 23:78-86, 2021.
- Galleri. Blood test for cancer screening: Galleri Test. https://www.galleri.com.
- Guo N, et al. Circulating tumor DNA detection in lung cancer patients before and after surgery. Sci Rep. 6:33519, 2016.
- Habli, Z, et al. Circulating Tumor Cell Detection Technologies and Clinical Utility: Challenges and Opportunities. Cancers (Basel). 12:1930, 2020.
- Klein EA, et al. Clinical validation of a targeted methylation-based multi-cancer early detection test using an independent validation set. Ann Oncol. 32:1167-1177, 2021.
- Mandel P, Metais P. Les acides nucléiques du plasma sanguin chez l'homme [Nuclear Acids In Human Blood Plasma]. Comptes rendus des seances de la Societe de biologie et de ses filiales. 142:241–243, 1948.

- Medina JE, et al. Cell-free DNA approaches for cancer early detection and interception. J Immunother Cancer. 11: e006013, 2023.
- Mullis K. The unusual origin of the polymerase chain reaction. Sci Am. 262:56-65, 1983.
- Nicholson BD, et al. Multi-cancer early detection test in symptomatic patients referred for cancer investigation in England and Wales (SYMPLIFY): a large-scale, observational cohort study. Lancet Oncol. 24:733-743, 2023.
- Schrag D, et al. Blood-based tests for multicancer early detection (PATHFINDER): a prospective cohort study. Lancet. 402:1251-1260, 2023.
- Sozzi G, et al. Analysis of circulating tumor DNA in plasma at diagnosis and during follow-up of lung cancer patients. Cancer Res. 61:4675-4678, 2001.
- Stroun M, et al. Isolation and characterization of DNA from the plasma of cancer patients. Eur J Cancer Clin Oncol. 23:707–712, 1987.
- Vogelstein B, et al. Circulating tumor DNA for noninvasive detection of colon cancer. Proc Natl Acad Sci U S A. 102:16368-16373, 2005.
- Vogelstein B, et al. Cancer genome landscapes. Science. 339:1546–1558, 2013.
- Wade R, et al. Multi-cancer early detection tests for general population screening: a systematic literature review. medRxiv, 2024.
  doi: https://doi.org/10.1101/2024.02.14.24302576.
- Wan JCM, et al. Genome-wide mutational signatures in low-coverage whole genome sequencing of cell-free DNA. Nat Commun. 13:4953, 2022.
- Xu S, et al. Circulating tumor DNA identified by targeted sequencing in advanced-stage non-small cell lung cancer patients. Cancer Lett. 370:324-331, 2016.

- Xu Z, et al. Frequent KIT mutations in human gastrointestinal stromal tumors. Sci Rep. 4:5907, 2014.
- Xu Z, et al. Genetic mutation analysis of human gastric adenocarcinomas using ion torrent sequencing platform. PLoS One. 9: e100442, 2014.

Chapter 7. Unveiling the Black Box of the Human Body

- Anupindi SA, et al. Diagnostic performance of whole-body MRI as a tool for cancer screening in children with genetic cancer-predisposing conditions. AJR Am J Roentgenol. 205:400-408, 2015.
- Basar Y, et al. Whole-body MRI for preventive health screening: management strategies and clinical implications. Eur J Radiol. 137:109584, 2021.
- Brown MA, Semelka RC. MRI: Basic Principles and Applications. John Wiley & Sons, 2011.
- Campbell-Washburn AE, et al. Opportunities in Interventional and Diagnostic Imaging by Using High-Performance Low-Field-Strength MRI. Radiology. 293:384-393, 2019.
- Consul N, et al. Li-Fraumeni syndrome and whole-body MRI screening: screening guidelines, imaging features, and impact on patient management. AJR Am J Roentgenol. 216:252-263, 2021.
- Damadian R. Tumor detection by nuclear magnetic resonance. Science. 171:1151-1153, 1971.
- Greer ML, Voss SD, States LJ. Pediatric cancer predisposition imaging: focus on whole-body MRI. Clin Cancer Res. 23: e6–e13. 2017.
- Hashemi RH, Bradley WG Jr. MRI: The Basics, 4th Edition, 2018.
- Hu, YS., Wu, CA., Lin, DC. et al. Applying ONCO-RADS to whole-body MRI cancer screening in a retrospective cohort of asymptomatic individuals. Cancer Imaging 24, 22 (2024). https://doi.org/10.1186/s40644-024-00665-z

- Kwee RM, Kwee TC. Whole-body MRI for preventive health screening: a systematic review of the literature. J Magn Reson Imaging. 50:1489-1503, 2019.
- Lauterbur PC. Image formation by induced local interactions: Examples of employing nuclear magnetic resonance. Nature. 242:190-191, 1973.
- Möllenhoff K, Oros-Peusquens AM, Shah NJ. Introduction to the basics of magnetic resonance imaging. Molecular Imaging in the Clinical Neurosciences, 75-98, 2012.
- Petralia G, et al. Whole-body magnetic resonance imaging (WB-MRI) for cancer screening: recommendations for use. Radiol Med. 126:1434–1450, 2021.
- Petralia G, et al. Oncologically relevant findings reporting and data system (ONCO-RADS): guidelines for the acquisition, interpretation, and reporting of whole-body MRI for cancer screening. Radiology. 299:494-507, 2021.
- Plenge E, et al. Super-resolution methods in MRI: can they improve the trade-off between resolution, signal-to-noise ratio, and acquisition time? Magn Reson Med. 68:1983-1993, 2012.
- Purcell EM, Torrey HC, Pound RV. Resonance absorption by nuclear moments in a solid. Phys Rev. 69:37-38, 1946.
- Purcell EM. Research in nuclear magnetism. Nobel Lecture, pp 219-231, 1952 from nobelprize.org.
- Rabi II. Space quantization in a gyrating magnetic field. Phys Rev. 51:652-654, 1937.
- Westbrook C. Handbook of MRI Technique, 5th Edition, 2021.
- Zugni F, et al. Whole-body magnetic resonance imaging (WB-MRI) for cancer screening in asymptomatic subjects of the general population: review and recommendations. Cancer Imaging. 20:34, 2020.

Chapter 8. Transforming Systemic Early Detection with AI

- Albarqouni S, et al. A federated learning approach for enhancing MRI diagnostics with artificial intelligence. Nat Mach Intell. 4:685–695, 2022.
- Castiglioni I, et al. AI applications to medical images: From machine learning to deep learning. Phys Med. 83:9-24, 2021.
- Epstein Z, et al. Art and the science of generative AI. Science. 380:1110-1111, 2023.
- Fritz B, Fritz J. Artificial intelligence for MRI diagnosis of joints: a scoping review of the current state-of-the-art of deep learning-based approaches. Skeletal Radiol. 51:315-329, 2022.
- Fui-Hoon Nah F, et al. Generative AI and ChatGPT: Applications, challenges, and AI-human collaboration. JITCAR. 25:277-304, 2023.
- GE HealthCare. Achieving greater connectivity in Radiology through digitization and AI. 2022. https://www.gehealthcare.com/insights/article/achieving-greater-connectivity-in-radiology-through-digitization-and-ai.
- GE HealthCare. Deep learning image reconstruction: Improving IQ and patient outcomes in radiology. 2023. https://www.gehealthcare.com/insights/article/deep-learning-image-reconstruction-improving-iq-and-patient-outcomes-in-radiology.
- Ginghina O, et al. Liquid Biopsy and Artificial Intelligence as Tools to Detect Signatures of Colorectal Malignancies: A Modern Approach in Patient's Stratification. Front Oncol. 12:856575, 2022.
- Goodfellow I, et al. Generative Adversarial Nets. Proc Int Conf Neural Inf Process Syst (NIPS 2014). pp. 2672–2680.
- Hajjo R, et al. Identification of tumor-specific MRI biomarkers using machine learning (ML). Diagnostics. 11:742, 2021.

- Kingma DP, Welling M. Auto-Encoding Variational Bayes. arXiv:1312.6114, 2013.
- Moser T, et al. Bridging biological cfDNA features and machine learning approaches. Trends Genet. 39:285-307, 2023.
- NVIDIA AI Platform. https://www.nvidia.com/en-us/ai-data-science/.
- NVIDIA Clara for Medical Imaging. https://www.nvidia.com/en-us/clara/medical-imaging/.
- Patil S, Shankar H. Transforming healthcare: harnessing the power of AI in the modern era. Int J Multidiscip Sci Arts. 2:60-70, 2023.
- Pinsky PF. Principles of cancer screening. Surg Clin North Am. 95:953-966, 2015.
- Post C, et al. Multicancer Early Detection Tests: An Overview of Early Results From Prospective Clinical Studies and Opportunities for Oncologists. JCO Oncol Pract. 19:1111-1115, 2023.
- Prorok PC, Kramer BS, Gohagan JK. Screening theory and study design: the basics. Cancer screening. CRC Press, 2021. pp. 29-53.
- Raschka S, Patterson J, Nolet C. Machine learning in python: Main developments and technology trends in data science, machine learning, and artificial intelligence. Information. 11:193, 2020.
- Rehman MHU, et al. Federated learning for medical imaging radiology. Br J Radiol. 96:20220890, 2023.
- Schrag D, et al. Blood-based tests for multicancer early detection (PATHFINDER): a prospective cohort study. Lancet. 402:1251-1260, 2023.
- Turing A. Computing Machinery and Intelligence. Mind. 59:433–460, 1950. doi: 10.1093/mind/LIX.236.433.
- Usui K, et al. Evaluation of motion artefact reduction depending on the artefacts' directions in head MRI using

conditional generative adversarial networks. Sci Rep. 13:8526, 2023.

- Vaswani A, et al. Attention is all you need. Adv Neural Inf Process Syst. 30, 2017.
- Vittone J, et al. A multi-cancer early detection blood test using machine learning detects early-stage cancers lacking USPSTF-recommended screening. NPJ Precis Oncol. 8:91, 2024.
- Wang HY, et al. Integrating Artificial Intelligence for Advancing Multiple-Cancer Early Detection via Serum Biomarkers: A Narrative Review. Cancers. 16:862, 2024.
- Zhang Y, et al. A GPU-based computational framework that bridges Neuron simulation and Artificial Intelligence. Nat Commun. 14:5798, 2023.

Chapter 9. Enhancing Accessibility and Equality with AI

- Chen Y, et al. AI-based reconstruction for fast MRI—a systematic review and meta-analysis. Proc IEEE. 110:224-245, 2022.
- Johnson PM, Recht MP, Knoll F. Improving the speed of MRI with artificial intelligence. Semin Musculoskelet Radiol. 24:12-20, 2020.
- Man C, et al. Deep learning enabled fast 3D brain MRI at 0.055 tesla. Sci Adv. 9:eadi9327, 2023.
- Shimron E, Perlman O. AI in MRI: Computational Frameworks for a Faster, Optimized, and Automated Imaging Workflow. Bioengineering. 10:492, 2023.
- Ueda, T, et al. Compressed sensing and deep learning reconstruction for women's pelvic MRI denoising: utility for improving image quality and examination time in routine clinical practice. European J of Radiology 134: 109430, 2021.
- Zhao Y, et al. Whole-body magnetic resonance imaging at 0.05 Tesla. Science. 384:eadm7168, 2024.

Chapter 10. The Dawn of a New Era of Systemic Early Detection

- Benford D, Bonar S. How City of Hope is leading the way in early cancer detection, prevention. 2024.
- Blumenthal D, Gumas E, Shah A. The Failing U.S. Health System. N Engl J Med. 2024 Oct 9. doi: 10.1056/NEJMp2410855. PMID: 39383455.
- Dana-Farber's Centers for Early Detection and Interception.
- Datta M, et al. Prevalence of Intracranial Aneurysms Identified by Screening a General Population in North America: Association with Lifestyle and Medical Risk Factors (P2-5.011). Neurology. 2024. https://doi.org/10.1212/WNL.0000000000205718.
- Enriquez J. In the U.S. Healthcare Industry, a Slow Shift toward Prevention. Sci Am, 2022.
- Gunja MZ, et al. U.S. Health Care from a Global Perspective, 2022: Accelerating Spending, Worsening Outcomes. Commonwealth Fund. 2023. https://www.commonwealthfund.org/publications/issue-briefs/2023/jan/us-health-care-global-perspective-2022.
- Handler R. Reflections on Stanford's Digital Health Summit. How Digital Technology Can Pave the Way for a New Era of Accessible, Personalized, and Preventive Healthcare. 2024.
- Hood L. How Technology, Big Data, and Systems Approaches Are Transforming Medicine. Res Technol Manag. 62:24–30, 2019.
- Jared G. Medical industry to move from 'sick' care to focus on 'health' care. https://talkbusiness.net/2023/05/medical-industry-to-move-from-sick-care-to-focus-on-health-care/.
- Laboratory Developed Tests. FDA.
- Medical Device Safety and the 510(k) Clearance Process. FDA.
- Ofman J. Early Detection: Key to Reducing Costs of Late-Stage Cancer, Grail. 2023. https://grail.com.

- Philipson TJ, et al. The aggregate value of cancer screenings in the United States: full potential value and value considering adherence. BMC Health Serv Res. 23:829, 2023.
- Premarket Approval (PMA). FDA. https://www.fda.gov/medical-devices/premarket-submissions-selecting-and-preparing-correct-submission/premarket-approval-pma.
- Prenuvo. From sick care to health care. https://www.prenuvo.com/blog/from-sick-care-to-health-care#:~:text=Our%20Current%20Sick%20Care%20Paradigm,their%20overall%20health%20and%20wellbeing.
- Schüssler-Fiorenza R, et al. A longitudinal big data approach for precision health. Nat Med. 25:792–804, 2019.
- WHO. Cancer. https://www.who.int/news-room/fact-sheets/detail/cancer.

Chapter 11. Individual-Driven Systemic Early Detection

- American Association for Cancer Research (AACR) Annual Meeting. Accelerated Aging May Increase the Risk of Early-onset Cancers in Younger Generations. 2024.
- American Cancer Society. History of Colonoscopy. 2020. https://www.cancer.org.
- Avantect-Early Cancer Detection. https://www.avantect.com/early-detection-of-pancreatic-cancer/
- BBC. Why age matters when it comes to cancer. 2024. https://www.bbc.com/future/article/20240209-how-cancer-risk-increases-with-age.
- Blackford AL, et al. Recent Trends in the Incidence and Survival of Stage 1A Pancreatic Cancer: A Surveillance, Epidemiology, and End Results Analysis. J Natl Cancer Inst. 112:1162–1169, 2020.

- Callister MEJ, de Koning HJ. Lung cancer screening in never-smokers: a balancing act. Lancet Respir Med. 12:93-94, 2024.
- Gunja MZ, Gumas ED, Williams RD II. U.S. Health Care from a Global Perspective, 2022: Accelerating Spending, Worsening Outcomes. Commonwealth Fund. 2023. https://www.commonwealthfund.org/publications/issue-briefs/2023/jan/us-health-care-global-perspective-2022.
- Kerpel-Fronius A, et al. Screening for Lung Cancer in Individuals Who Never Smoked: An International Association for the Study of Lung Cancer Early Detection and Screening Committee Report. J Thorac Oncol. 17:56-66, 2022.
- Laconi E, Marongiu F, DeGregori J. Cancer as a disease of old age: changing mutational and microenvironmental landscapes. Br J Cancer. 122:943–952, 2020. https://doi.org/10.1038/s41416-019-0721-1.
- Lagasse J. US spends most on healthcare, has worst outcomes, finds Commonwealth Fund. Healthcare Finance. 2023. https://www.healthcarefinancenews.com/news/us-spends-most-healthcare-has-worst-outcomes-finds-commonwealth-fund.
- OECD Health Statistics. 2022. https://www.oecd-ilibrary.org/social-issues-migration-health/data/oecd-health-statistics_health-data-en
- Rex DK, et al. Colorectal Cancer Screening: Recommendations for Physicians and Patients. Am J Gastroenterol. 112:101-120, 2017.
- Schrag D, et al. Blood-based tests for multicancer early detection (PATHFINDER): a prospective cohort study. Lancet. 402:1251-1260, 2023.
- Winawer SJ, et al. Prevention of Colorectal Cancer by Colonoscopic Polypectomy. N Engl J Med. 329:1977-1981, 1993.

- Wolff WI, Shinya H. Polypectomy via the Fiberoptic Colonoscope: Removal of Neoplasms Beyond the Reach of the Sigmoidoscope. N Engl J Med. 288:329-332, 1973.

ACKNOWLEDGMENTS

I would like to express my heartfelt gratitude to all those who have made the writing of this book possible. My most profound appreciation goes to the over one hundred talented and dedicated graduate students, post-doctoral fellows, physicians, visiting scientists, and technicians who have worked in my laboratory over the past thirty years. Their relentless pursuit of innovative cancer therapies, preventive cancer vaccines, and ctDNA detection tests has been crucial to our progress.

I am profoundly thankful to the physicians and researchers who have partnered with me to develop and translate innovative approaches into clinical studies. Notable collaborators and supporters include Professor Frank Torti, MD, Professor Malcolm Brenner, MD, PhD, Professor Helen Heslop, MD, Professor Cliona Rooney, PhD, Professor Hu Chen, MD, Dr. Fang Hu, MD, Professor Jun Zhu, MD, PhD, Dr. Nancy T. Chang, PhD, and Dr. Gerald Chan, PhD, whose contributions have been invaluable in advancing our cancer therapies and detection. I am grateful for the mentorship and support of Professor Richard Compans, Professor Wayne Marasco, and Professor William Haseltine.

I also extend my gratitude to Professor Jun Wang, MD, Professor Jun Chen, MD, Dr. Tao Zhao, MD, and Mr. Rong Shi for their collaboration in the development of blood ctDNA tests. I appreciate the many other physicians and researchers not individually mentioned here for their collaboration and contributions.

Furthermore, I wish to acknowledge Professor Martin Kast, PhD, Professor James Ou, PhD, Professor Rongfu Wang, PhD, Professor Andre Ouellette, PhD, Professor Zhi Wang, MD, Professor Pinghui Feng, PhD, Professor Shaun Zhang, MD, PhD, Dr. Naimin Wei, MD, PhD, Dr. Yu Geng, MD, Professor Gutian Xiao, PhD, Professor Julia Qu, PhD, Associate Professor Joseph R. Landolph, Jr., PhD, Mrs. Susan Ou and many others for their insightful critiques and discussions, which have greatly enhanced this manuscript.

Finally, I am deeply grateful to my wife, Dr. Fiona X. Huang, for her longstanding collaboration in developing cancer immunotherapy and for her critical insights on this manuscript, as well as to my daughter, Kat Chen, for her thoughtful review and comments.

INDEX

N

O